NO ONE WANTS TO FEEL LIMITED BY BACK PAIN

Having a bad back need not prevent you from doing all the things you love to do or stop you from trying new ones. In this informative guide, Dr. Leon Root, a renowned orthopedic surgeon and co-author of the best-selling *Oh, My Aching Back,* offers invaluable advice that will keep you moving and keep you pain-free. This comprehensive book also includes tips on how to perform regular activities so as not to injure or strain your back, as well as a series of exercises that really work. The best news is that with Dr. Root's advice and recommendations for sports, sex and all kinds of everyday living, aching backs can become a thing of the past.

NO MORE
ACHING
B A C K

NO MORE ACHING BACK

Dr. Root's Fifteen-Minute-a-Day Program for a Healthy Back

LEON ROOT, M.D.

Illustrations by Elisa Root

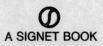

A SIGNET BOOK

SIGNET
Published by New American Library, a division of
Penguin Putnam Inc., 375 Hudson Street,
New York, New York 10014, U.S.A.
Penguin Books Ltd, 27 Wrights Lane,
London W8 5TZ, England
Penguin Books Australia Ltd, Ringwood,
Victoria, Australia
Penguin Books Canada Ltd, 10 Alcorn Avenue,
Toronto, Ontario, Canada M4V 3B2
Penguin Books (N.Z.) Ltd, 182–190 Wairau Road,
Auckland 10, New Zealand

Penguin Books Ltd, Registered Offices:
Harmondsworth, Middlesex, England

Published by Signet, an imprint of New American Library,
a division of Penguin Books USA Inc. This is an authorized reprint
of a hardcover edition published by Villard Books, a division of
Random House, Inc. The hardcover edition was published simultaneously
in Canada by Random House of Canada Limited, Toronto.

First Signet Printing, November 1991

17   16   15   14

Ⓟ REGISTERED TRADEMARK—MARCA REGISTRADA

Printed in the United States of America

NOTE TO THE READER
The ideas, procedures, and suggestions contained in this book are not intended as a
substitute for consulting with your physician. All matters regarding your health require medical supervision.

To all my patients,
whose experiences are the foundation
of this book

Preface

Science is the search for knowledge. This eternal quest to advance the betterment of mankind does not stop with a new discovery or method, but rather increases the drive for further improvements in the way we do things. It is especially true with medicine, the science most intimately concerned with the functioning of the human body. Doctors and researchers are constantly updating the body of knowledge concerned with making life more comfortable and enjoyable for us. This is equally true for the area of the body, the back, that continues to be a source of major discomfort to millions of sufferers each year. This book updates my previous writings and contains the most recent and comprehensive information available on the diagnosis and treatment of back problems.

Acknowledgments

This book has been a labor of love supported and enhanced by my family. My wife, Paula, and our children, Matthew and Lili, allowed me time to write on weekends, time which I usually reserve for them. Their love and good humor made work pleasurable and the results worthwhile.

I am endebted to my brother, Norman Root, who spent numerous hours reviewing my manuscript. His advice and counsel were invaluable in the organization of the material and in making certain that my thoughts and concepts would be clear to you, my readers. Since our childhood days, he has inspired me to new levels of achievement.

The wonderful illustrations were done by my niece, Elisa Root. I took full advantage of her artistic talents and excellent concepts to provide you with illustrations that would help to explain my message and the exercise programs.

There are two people outside my family whom I also wish to acknowledge and thank: my editor, Diane Reverand, whose encouragement and sage advice made the whole process enjoyable and educational, and my loyal and industrious secretary, Norma Bonaiuto, who worked all those extra early-morning and late-night hours typing the manuscript over and over again.

Without the help and support of these wonderful people, this book would not have been possible.

Leon Root

Contents

List of Illustrations

List of Exercises

Introduction

You are probably reading this book because you have personally experienced a problem with your back, or have been close to someone who has had a bad experience with his or her back. In any case, you are concerned about avoiding and preventing the debilitating experience of being laid up with a bad back. Your concern is well founded.

Despite all medical efforts, back problems continue to plague mankind. In the United States, approximately 80 million people have or are suffering from back pain. The U.S. government reports that $25 billion is spent each year on health care for these people. At a recent meeting of the American Academy of Orthopaedic Surgeons, there were nearly one hundred papers, exhibits, instructional courses, and seminars that dealt solely with low-back pain.

Back pain is ubiquitous; it knows no boundaries and is seen in every walk of life. President John F. Kennedy had surgery for his back, and his use of a rocking chair to ease his pain became famous. Joe Montana, the quarterback for the San Francisco 49ers, astounded the world by having surgery for a herniated disk in his lower back and returning to full contact in eight weeks. A famous conductor does his back exercises every day in order to stand on the podium and wave his baton at the orchestra. Every day I see a multitude of secretaries, teachers, executives, construction workers, lawyers, and even doctors—not to mention pregnant women, actors and actresses, writers, and computer specialists—all of whom complain about pain in their backs. The cause of almost all of these people's pain is mechanical. In other words, their back problems do not originate from a sickness or disease, but rather a problem with the muscles, ligaments, intervertebral disks, and bones that are the essential parts of the spinal structure.

A question that always arises is whether or not back pain is a new problem for man. Did the farmers, laborers, artisans, soldiers, and professional people of the past experience the same magnitude of back problems as modern man does? Or is something new happening, which is perhaps linked to the greater emotional and physical stress associated with disruptions in people's habits in this changing world? These questions are difficult to answer because we do not have available data to make scientific comparisons.

We do know that back pain is not new. Indeed, doctors, faith healers, surgeons, chiropractors, and osteopaths have applied various skills to relieve the pain of these sufferers for centuries. In all cases, however, treatment followed pain. Until fairly recently in this century, there was little concentration on how to prevent back pain; most efforts were directed toward relieving it once it occurs. The sad truth is that although most treatment is successful in relieving the pain, back attacks are usually recurrent.

Part of the problem is that different factors can cause back pain. We know that back problems seem to run in some families, so perhaps hereditary aspects play a role. For years, the fact that man has stood erect, rather than on all four limbs, has been considered a major cause of stress for the lower back. However, even four-legged animals like the dachshund develop slipped disks in their spines.

Research to determine the effects of lifting and bending on the spine is done at dozens of medical centers throughout the world. The Volvo car makers, with the guidance of orthopedic surgeons, have tested the effect that car seats have upon the back. Back schools have proliferated like mushrooms across the country. Sports medicine centers and local Y's advertise exercise programs for back sufferers and for those who wish to avoid these perplexing and sometimes agonizing problems. We are immersed in a sea of information, much of it incomplete, some of it contradictory, and most of it confusing.

After almost thirty years of treating and studying patients with back problems and having to deal with my own back problems, I feel that I can help people, not only to get over their back pain, but to avoid it in the first place. In this book, I shall show you how to do both. But before you can embark on a program for a healthy back, you must be aware of what constitutes a healthy back.

This book is addressed to you, the reader, as if you are a patient with a back problem coming to my office for the first time. During the course of this office visit, I will describe how I conduct an examination and why I perform certain tests. Next I will tell you about the structure of the back and how it functions, using minimal but necessary medical terminology. This will be followed by an alarming section on what can go wrong with your back. But don't worry, ensuing sections describe how back prolems are identified and treated, and offer short- and long-term solutions for alleviating and avoiding back pain. Next in order are a number of helpful hints on the kinds of physical activities in which back-conscious people can engage, including sex, sports, and exercises. Last but not least, I will describe and illustrate the exercise program I have developed to strengthen and protect your back.

Does that seem like a tall order? It is, but don't be discouraged. Contrary to what you may be thinking, I will not be tedious or overly technical, as you will discover as you read along. However, there is one essential point that I must make now (and I shall repeat it many times in this book): *The only one who can ultimately make your back better is you.*

It is not as hard to do as it may sound. Experience has shown that 90 percent of the people with back pain get better with time, even without any treatment. The crucial issue is to prevent it from occurring again and again, which is the distressing aspect of a low-back problem. I hope I have stimulated your interest. Now, read on and find out what you need to know about back pain and how to have a healthy back. *You* can achieve that goal. Good luck and good reading.

LEON ROOT, M.D.
January 1, 1990

1. The Office Visit

Welcome to my office. I am sorry we have to meet under these circumstances, which may have you suffering from back pain. In the course of my examination, I may use some technical terms that you will not understand. Following the examination, I hope the terms will become clear as I describe the structure of the back and how it functions.

The objective of an examination is to identify or diagnose what is wrong with your back. There is an established logical sequence of events that leads to a diagnosis. First and foremost is a complete history of the complaint. The famous internist Sir William Osler wrote that if you listen carefully to the patient, the patient will tell you what is wrong with him or her. Next is the physical examination, with emphasis upon back mechanics, movements, and neurocirculatory evaluation, followed by X-rays and blood tests as indicated by history or physical examination.

HISTORY OF COMPLAINTS AND
PHYSICAL EXAMINATION

The first time you go to a specialist's office is often an anxiety-provoking experience. You wonder if the doctor will be sympathetic and understanding, and whether the doctor's examination will provoke additional pain. Will there be time for discussion? Will explanations be given so that you can understand what is wrong? And finally, there is always the underlying fear that the diagnosis will be very serious and require surgery; or worse, what if it is cancer? These are all normal thoughts and reactions as you come through the office door. Some people are nervous and others are quite calm, but you are approaching a new experience, and that always promotes a degree of apprehension. I cannot alleviate that feeling entirely, but for the most part you can rest assured that I am here to listen and help you. So enter the office with a confident attitude.

In addition to confidence, bring along all X-rays that have been done of your back and whatever recent laboratory blood tests were performed. If you have written reports from other doctors regarding your general health or even consultations with other specialists with regard to your back, bring them along as well. Remember that a doctor is like a detective; he assembles as many clues as he can get that prove "culpability" and then arrests the guilty party—actually innocent until proven guilty. At any rate, the more information, both old and new, that I have, the better able I will be to arrive at the right diagnosis and thus institute the right treatment for your aching back.

Also come prepared to give a thorough and sequential history of your complaints. Try to remember the first time you had back pain and how it occurred. It is important to know if the pain is localized in your lower back or radiates down the leg into your foot. Knowing where the pain is and how far it travels provides important clues to its cause. Try to describe the pain in such words as "nagging, toothache, sharp, knifelike, burning, pins and needles, and tingling." All of these have special significance for me.

Is your pain relieved by lying down, and if so, in what position are you most comfortable in bed? Is your pain worse with sitting? Do coughing or sneezing increase your symptoms? Most of the time patients just think of the pain itself without trying to focus upon what affects it. Is your pain getting worse? Are the pains more intense? Are attacks coming more frequently and lasting longer? Are the pains that were initially only in your back now radiating or traveling into your legs, or radiating around to the stomach or groin area?

If you categorize your pain symptoms, you are providing very important information. I shall ask you about past treatments for your back or leg. I shall want to know what medicines you have taken and how effective or ineffective they have been. If you have been to a chiropractor, osteopath, physical therapist, masseur/masseuse, or an acupuncturist, I should know that, and whether or not they helped (probably not enough, or you wouldn't be in my office).

Do hot or cold applications help? The age-old question of whether to apply heat or ice is still always asked. The answer is both. Actually there are specific indications for hot or cold applications, but neither provides more than temporary relief or comfort.

After asking these specific questions relating to pain, I will want to obtain some general information about your health and activities. Have you ever had any serious illnesses, operations, other joint problems, or do you have any allergies to medicines? I shall inquire about the stresses of your everyday physical activities and emotional reactions. Do you have a stressful or physically demanding job? Are you taking care of a house and children and participating in a driving pool three days a week? Do you sit a lot or travel long distances? Are you getting any exercise besides walking up and down the stairs several times a day? Remember, being on your feet all day, running from a house to the car, or from your office to another office, or standing behind a counter serving people, or driving a truck or a cab, are not exercise but work. Work is necessary, and I hope pleasant and rewarding for you, but work, unless you are a professional athlete or aerobics teacher, is not necessarily exercise. At least not the kind that improves your stamina and helps your back. Are you a weekend athlete? Do you do any regular exercises, such as yoga, calisthenics, or aerobics?

The next series of questions will involve your social habits. How much alcohol do you drink? Are you a smoker? (Several epidemiological studies have shown a strong association between cigarette smoking and low-back pain as well as sciatica and even osteoporosis.)

Are you married, and are you happy at home? How do you handle stress? These are personal questions coming from a stranger across the desk, but I am trying to learn as much about you as I can in order to have as complete a picture of you as possible in a relatively short time.

Besides learning about you, I will want to know about your family's medical history. Although there is no evidence to support a genetic inheritance of back pain in the narrow context, there is significant increased prevalence of back and disk problems in relatives of patients with these problems. Actually that information could also be important for your children. If you have back problems, encourage them at an early age to develop good postural habits and other healthful programs so that they can avoid similar problems.

After obtaining the history of your pain, I will then examine you. Each doctor has his own particular system of examining a patient with low-back pain. I shall describe how I perform that examination in order to give you an overall view of the procedure. I shall also explain the significance of particular findings during the examination. Before I begin the discussion, however, it's important to point out that one single finding during an examination does not establish the diagnosis. For example, someone who has leg pain with limited ability to raise his/her leg may not necessarily have a herniated disk, although that is a common symptom of herniated disks. It is the aggregation of the clues and facts from the history and physical findings that enables the doctor to come to a logical and definitive diagnosis.

Naturally you have to undress completely for a back examination. For modesty, you'll wear a gown that opens in the back or a pair of gym-type shorts. I shall ask you to stand, and observe your posture.

The positions of your shoulders and your spine are among the first clues to the health of your back. Are you round-shouldered? Do you have an increased lordosis (swayback)? Is your spine straight, or does it curve to the side as if scoliosis is present? I will ask you to bend forward, backward, sideways, and to twist your trunk to either side to determine the suppleness of your spine. A decrease in spinal flexibility can be indicative of a back problem. A stiff back with limited range of motion can be due to, among other causes, muscle spasms, slipped disk, or inflammation of the spine. During this study of your body's flexibility, I also will be watching to see if you have pain associated with any particular movements.

Pains with certain movements can be related to specific problems. For instance, someone with a herniated disk may experience sciatic pain when bending to the side, whereas sufferers from spinal stenosis (narrowing of the spinal canal) may feel more comfortable bending forward and have pain if they attempt to bend backward. Again, let me emphasize that the result of one test alone does not constitute a diagnosis. Several confirmatory findings on examination are necessary to identify the problem.

The need for corroboration of symptoms is especially important because many times various signs or findings are overlapping. A herniated disk may resemble spinal stenosis or vice versa. In fact, both may exist at the same time. Back spasms may limit mobility of your back on the basis of just a muscle problem or in conjunction with a herniated disk or spinal stenosis. "One swallow does not make a spring," and one positive aspect of the examination does not make a diagnosis.

Next I will ask you to walk in a normal fashion. I want to see if you walk with a limp or experience any weakness or pain with walking. I will also look at the configuration of your feet. Do you have flat feet? Do you have a high arch? Do you have bunions? Feet may not be the cause of back pains, but often they may mirror a general body condition that could have an effect upon your back or vice versa. Some back abnormalities may be reflected in your feet. I may ask you to walk on your toes (like a ballerina) or on your heels (like a duck) in order to detect weakness or coordination problems. While you are still standing, I may ask you to hop on one leg or even to jar down hard on your heels.

Now back to the examination. Until now, I have simply looked without touching. Essentially I have studied the movements of your spine to determine which are limited and which are painful.

Following the standing evaluation, I'll ask you to sit on the edge of the examining table. In this position, with your knees bent over the edge of the table, I shall test your knee and ankle reflexes. I will also have you move your legs back and forth and once again examine your feet. Next I'll ask you to lie on your back on the examining table, and I shall take measurements of your legs to see if they are of equal length, and I also shall measure the girth or size of your thighs and calves, again to determine if they are equal.

Leg-length differences rarely cause back pain. This was dramatically brought to my attention some years ago when I examined an older gentleman who had had an infection of his hip in childhood that resulted in a shortening of that leg by almost two inches. Not only had he never experienced back pain (in spite of being an avid walker and hiker), but he always thought his limp was due to the hip abnormality and not to his short leg. However, his leg-length discrepancy was present from childhood, and his body had adapted to it. People who develop leg-length differences in later life may not be so fortunate, and their backs may not adjust to the new stresses and strains, but the difference in leg length is easily compensated by a lift on the shoe of the short leg.

A small difference in the size of the thighs or calves is also generally not significant, especially if someone is strongly dominant right- or left-handed. Conversely, if there is *atrophy,* or wasting of a thigh or calf muscle related to disuse or lack of use of the muscle because of pain, or if the nerve to the muscle is being compromised (particularly by a herniated disk), the difference in size becomes significant. It is also important to record these measurements for future reference to document improvement or progression of the problem.

While you are lying down, I will complete the remainder of the neurological examination. I have already tested your deep tendon reflexes (knee and ankle reflexes). Now, I shall check the sensation in your legs and lower body. Many people complain of numbness in their legs or toes, yet when tested they perceive sensation in an almost normal fashion. It is important to distinguish between those feelings and the actual loss of sensation to a particular area. A real or true loss of sensation reflects damage or compression of the nerve. Each region of the skin is supplied by a specific nerve. For example, the S1 nerve root supplies the outer border of the foot (the side of the foot with the little toe); the L5 nerve root supplies the outer side of the calf, and the inner side of the foot and the big toe. With this specificity, one can determine which nerve root is involved. Sensation is generally tested with a sharp object like a pin or the edge of a key. Usually testing is not painful, but is in a sense "scratchy."

Not only does sensation relate to specific nerve roots, but so does muscle strength. As with the skin, each muscle in your leg is supplied by a specific nerve or nerves. Indeed, some muscles have more than one nerve supplying them. In testing for muscle weakness, I shall ask you to hold your foot or leg in a certain way and resist my attempts to change the position. For instance, I may ask that you hold your great toe up, pointed toward your face. Then I shall test the muscle by trying to pull your toe downward. A normal muscle will strongly resist my pressure. If it is weak, I will be able to bring the toe downward with minimal difficulty. If it is very weak, the position change will be easy. Weakness of great-toe extension (that is, lifting it toward your face) indicates a problem with the L5 nerve root. On the other hand (or should I say, other foot?), weakness of flexion or pushing the great toe downward implicates the S1 nerve root. Several muscles in the ankles, knees, and hips are similarly tested, and any loss of muscle strength is noted. The combination of decreased reflexes, loss of sensation, muscle weakness, and atrophy of thigh or calf are indicative of a problem with the nerve root, and in most instances is due to pressure on the nerve by a herniated disk.

Evaluation of the circulation to your legs is done by checking the condition of the skin and feeling for the pulses in your feet. Strong pulses—that is, pulses that are easily felt—generally mean that a good supply of blood is flowing through your legs. If there is a blockage to blood flow higher up the leg, the pulses will be absent or difficult to feel. Older people with arteriosclerosis (narrowing of the blood vessels) may also have poor pulses in their feet. Swelling of the ankles or feet may be indicative of a general circulatory problem, especially if the swelling is in both feet.

Inflammation of the veins in the calves or thighs (phlebitis) can cause leg pains that mimic sciatica. However, in these cases, the calf is swollen, hard, and tender to touch, whereas with sciatica the calf is soft and nontender. Am I making this too complicated? Well, diagnosing back symptoms and sciatica is not simple, because circulatory problems and other conditions can also cause pains in the back and legs. That is why it is important to perform a very thorough examination.

Let us continue with the exam. You are still on your back, resting comfortably, I hope. If lying flat on your back is painful, as it is with many patients who suffer from a herniated disk, I shall ask you to keep your knees bent. This position relaxes tension on your sciatic nerve and relieves pain. You may have discovered this position on your own.

Straight-leg raising is a standard maneuver with all back patients. Keeping your knee straight, I will slowly lift the foot and leg from the table, going as high as possible before pain or tightness of the hamstrings limits the motion. If your sciatic nerve is under tension from a herniated disk, the range of elevation is markedly restricted. If the nerve is not under tension, the leg can be lifted easily to 70 or 80 degrees or almost straight up. This test is often done with the hip bent and knee bent to 90 degrees. Keeping the hip bent, the leg is gradually straightened. Again, the decreased ability to straighten the knee is dependent upon the tension on the sciatic nerve or tightness of the hamstrings. If the nerve is under tension, pain occurs in the leg and often the buttocks as well. If hamstring tightness limits motion, the range will be limited but not painful.

Tight hamstring muscles are very frequently associated with back problems. People who have "loose" or stretched-out hamstrings rarely have problems with their lower back. These individuals can bend over with their knees straight and place their palms upon the floor. But if you have tight hamstrings, when you bend forward with your knees straight, you are fortunate if your fingertips extend below your knees. The same is true of straight-leg raising. If your hamstrings are not tight (and you don't have sciatic-nerve involvement), you should be able to raise your leg 90 degrees. If your hamstrings are tight, you may only reach 60 degrees. Tight hamstrings alone are not painful. However, people with tight hamstrings are very prone to have back problems. The tight hamstrings limit normal pelvic motions, which in turn cause a great deal of additional strain on the lower back. Incidentally, until those hamstrings are properly stretched and lengthened, your back problems are likely to recur.

The next few tests are done to evaluate your lower-back and hip motion. I shall bend your hips and knees and bring your thighs toward your chest. If you do not have lumbar muscle spasm, this position is usually comfortable. Patients who have a herniated disk often find this position to be relaxing. However, if muscle spasms are present in your lower back, this movement will be limited and painful.

Testing the movement of the hip joints is carried out by rolling the hips in and out and extending them with one thigh pressed against your chest and the other leg brought to the table. If you have normal hip joints, these movements are painless. However, if osteoarthritis or some other problem affecting the hip is present, then the motions may be painful and limited. If the hip joint moves freely without pain, then the pain you have been experiencing is not related to the hip. However, if these movements are restricted and painful, then there is a strong possibility that your pain is coming from the hip. Some patients have both back and hip problems, in which case both conditions must be treated in order to relieve their pain.

With this part of the examination completed, it is time to turn onto your stomach. While you're in this "prone" position, I shall palpate or touch your spine. At first I'll use light pressure, and then gradually heavy pressure. I'll start from the neck and work down to the coccyx area. I shall thump along your spine with the side of my hand. I'll also thump over the areas of your kidneys to see if they are sensitive.

I'll press along the crest of your pelvic bones. These maneuvers are used to discover "sore" or tender spots in the back, and are further attempts to pinpoint the source of your pain. Because the spinal bones and nerves are covered by thick muscles, it is difficult to feel or palpate the bones and nerves directly. The spinous processes, which project backward and are easily palpated under the skin, are rarely ever the source of pain. However, deep pressure may elicit pain over an inflamed facet joint or an injured ligament or a bruised muscle. Pressing on your lower back with the palm of my hand pushes your lower spine forward; this maneuver will produce pain in your back and leg if a herniated disk is pressed against the nerve root.

An early sign of a compromised S1 nerve root is loss of muscle tone in the buttocks on the involved side. If you clench (voluntarily contract) your buttocks together so that they are made "hard" (like flexing any muscle), each buttock should feel firm and solid. If one side is "softer" than the other, it indicates a decrease in muscle tone, which may be due to a herniated disk.

By now, you are probably aware that during the examination I compare one side to the other—muscle strength, sensation, straight-leg raising, buttock tone, etc. Since symptoms are one-sided in the majority of cases, especially with disk herniations, it is important to compare one side to the other to determine differences.

While you are still in the prone position, I shall have you lift up your legs, one at a time, from your hips, keeping the knee straight. A second test will require you to raise your head and shoulders with your hands behind your back. These maneuvers stress the lower-back region and the muscles in the lower back and buttocks. Pain with these tests is indicative of low-back problems. If the pain radiates into the leg, that is another sign of a herniated disk or spinal stenosis.

A rectal or vaginal examination is important in evaluating back pain. If the patient has had a recent rectal or vaginal examination done by an internist or gynecologist, it is not necessary to repeat the examination. However, if such an exam has not been done recently, a rectal examination is essential. I refer my female patients to their gynecologist for the vaginal examination.

Palpation of the abdomen and listening to the chest and lungs are done whenever symptoms or findings are suspicious for problems in these areas.

The basic examination is now completed. Certain other tests may be done, depending upon what I found during the examination. Each doctor has his/her own way of proceeding with the examination. I have described my method of examination and have given you a brief interpretation of what the various tests mean. Hopefully, if you ever have to see a doctor for your back, this brief explanation will ease the anxiety that the upcoming visit may present.

A brief summary may help you place the examination in a better perspective. First, I checked the overall structure and posture of your back and watched you walk. I observed the range of motion of your spine. I evaluated the neurocirculatory status of your legs. I checked for sciatic-nerve tension with straight-leg raising. I tested motions of your hips and lower back. While you were on your stomach, I pressed along your back to evaluate the spine and associated structures. I may also have done a rectal examination.

After obtaining your history and conducting the physical examination, I am now able to put all the "facts" together and come up with a diagnosis and a treatment program for your problem. Sometimes this can be formulated without any further tests, but often X-rays and blood tests are needed to verify the diagnosis before treatment can be carried out. Later I will tell you about the various tests that are available to help make a correct diagnosis. In the next chapter, I am going to describe the structure of the back and explain some of the medical terms that I have been using so that you will have a better understanding of how the back functions.

2. How Your Back Works

The prospect of reading a chapter on the human anatomy may seem onerous, but I have no intention of overwhelming you with the anatomy of the back. On the other hand, some basic knowledge of the structures of the spine and how it works is essential for the understanding of what can go wrong and what you can do to correct the problems. After all, if you do not know how the bolts hold the wheel onto your car, you would not be able to fix a flat. The anatomy of the back is obviously more complex than that.

Everyone knows that the spine extends from the base of the skull to the pelvis, that it consists of bones, muscles, and disks, and that the spinal cord and its nerves are inside these bones. You know that the spine has mobility because you can bend and twist and these movements occur throughout your spine. Names are given to different areas of the spine. The upper part of the back is the neck or *cervical* spine. The area behind the ribs is called the *dorsal* or *thoracic* spine. The area in the lower part of the back, between the ribs and the pelvis, is known as the *lumbar* spine. The very lower parts are the *sacrum* and *coccyx*. These regions can be easily identified on a skeleton or on your own back.

15

FIGURE OF SPINE #1

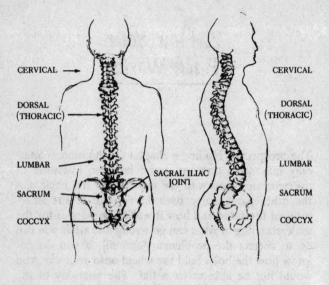

CERVICAL →

DORSAL (THORACIC) →

LUMBAR →

SACRAL ILIAC JOINT

SACRUM →

COCCYX →

CERVICAL

DORSAL (THORACIC)

LUMBAR

SACRUM

COCCYX

As seen in Figure 1, the spinal column is not a long, solid bone. Rather, it is a series of individual bone blocks stacked one upon the other. We know these plurally as the *vertebrae;* singularly, *vertebra*. Contrary to popular belief, the vertebral bone is not shaped like a bagel with a hole in the middle. Since one picture is worth a thousand words, the structure is best described by the diagram on page 17.

Note that one side of the vertebra is rounded and the other side irregular, with several projections. The opening behind the round portion in conjunction with the vertebrae above and below form a continuous canal through which pass the spinal cord and nerve roots. Ligaments are strong bands of tissue that help

THE FIVE LUMBAR VERTEBRAE #2

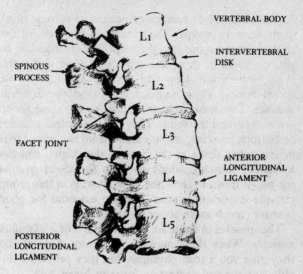

VERTEBRAL BODY

INTERVERTEBRAL DISK

SPINOUS PROCESS

FACET JOINT

ANTERIOR LONGITUDINAL LIGAMENT

POSTERIOR LONGITUDINAL LIGAMENT

L1

L2

L3

L4

L5

hold the bones together. The disks between the blocks of bones, (the famous intervertebral disks that can be the cause of many back problems) act as shock absorbers and allow a small amount of motion to occur between each bone. Small joints on either side of the back of the vertebral bodies also connect the bones to each other. These are called *facet joints*. Intertwining and overlapping the entire skeletal structure and stretching from the head to the knees are muscles that connect to and control the movements of the spine. Muscle movement in turn is stimulated by the extensive nerve network in response to commands from the brain reacting to the environment. Now that is your first anatomy lesson. Not too difficult. Let's take a closer look, first from the outside.

17

Muscles

Rather than try to remember dozens of names, think of muscles as groups. The groups on the back of the spine hold the spine straight when you are standing or sitting. Some of these are superficial (just under the skin), others are deep and directly attached to the spinal bones. These muscles are called the *extensor* muscles. Two other sets of muscles in this same group are also behind the spine. They are the *gluteus* muscles or buttock muscles, which extend from the upper part of the pelvis down to the back of the thighs, and the *hamstring* muscles, which go from the lower part of the pelvis down to the knee. The muscles in this group provide important support and are essential for good posture (much more about posture later).

The muscles in front are your stomach or *abdominal* muscles. When these muscles are strong, not only do they give you a trim physique, but they provide valuable support and protection for your lower back.

Finally there are the muscles that lie deep inside your body against the sides of your spine (just to satisfy your curiosity, they are known as the *iliopsoas* and *quadratus lumborum* muscles). Now what I want you to have in mind is a concept of your spine with many movable segments being supported in the back, in the front, and on the sides by special groups of muscles. Each set is important, and they all work together to provide the motion and protection that are essential to your back. If one set of muscles is weak and fails to do its job, the entire system can lean off balance. Just imagine a tripod trying to stand on only two of its legs! Thus, lesson one teaches that all three muscle groups must be strong and balanced in order to prevent unnatural movements in the spine that could really stress those connecting ligaments, intervertebral disks, and facet joints. It is these same muscles that are responsible for your ability to stand up straight and maintain good posture.

Bones

The bony construction of the spine is unique. In fact, species of animals are defined by the absence or presence of a *vertebral column.* Mammals, birds, and reptiles are all vertebrate, because they all have a spinal column consisting of separate bones attached to each other by ligaments and intervertebral disks with a spinal cord running through these bones. On the other hand, insects and crustaceans such as shrimp are known as *invertebrate,* because they do not have a backbone. The spinal column, or backbone, provides the support that enables us to stand upright with our heads over our pelvis, allows motion between each segment, and finally protects the spinal cord and nerves that connect your limbs to your brain.

The vertebral bone can be divided into front and back parts. In the front is the rounded, thick, solid bone whose major function is support. (See Figure 3.) The posterior portion consists of a space or canal created by a bony roof with a large posterior projection that is known as the *spinous process.* Bones project from either side of the back of the body (the *transverse processes).* The spinal canal forms the protective shell for the spinal cord. Muscles attach to the back and sides of the vertebral bones. Each vertebral body is equipped with four small, saucerlike structures (two on either side, top and bottom). The two on the top interface with the two on the bottom of the vertebra above. The two on the bottom interface with the two on the top of the vertebra below. This meeting of the superior and inferior facets forms a joint on either

VERTEBRAL BODY #3

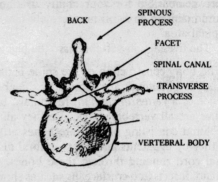

BACK

SPINOUS PROCESS

FACET

SPINAL CANAL

TRANSVERSE PROCESS

VERTEBRAL BODY

FRONT

side of the vertebral bodies at each level. These joints, the facet joints, control motion between each vertebral segment. If these were not present, your spine would probably roll around in any direction, with minimal restraint and, needless to say, harm to your back. However, as you will learn later, excessive stress on this restraining function can be a source of back pain.

Although the vertebral bones are similar in appearance and readily recognizable, bones from different parts of the spine have specific characteristics. The seven cervical or neck vertebrae are smaller than the ones below; after all, they only have to support the weight of the head. The first and second vertebrae (known as the *atlas* and *axis*) are specially adapted to connect with the base of the skull and to provide a wide range of movement from nodding "yes" to swinging the head for "no." How would you ever hold your telephone against your shoulder if you could not lean your head to the side? The dorsal or thoracic vertebrae (twelve of these) have special sites for the attachments of the ribs (twelve on each side). Because of the encasing affect of the ribs, very little movement occurs between each of these vertebrae. Disk herniation (ruptured or slipped disks) is extremely rare in the dorsal-spinal area.

The five lumbar vertebrae are the biggest and strongest of all the vertebral bones. They support the weight of the upper body and yet provide mobility. These bones and the disks between them take the greatest stress. The lower down the lumbar spine, the greater will be that stress; 95 percent of all disk problems in the entire spine occur in the lowest portions of the movable spine L4–L5 and L5–S1. (The *L* refers to lumbar, and the number identifies the site of the vertebra. The five vertebrae in the lumbar region are numbered 1 through 5, starting from the top. The vertebrae in the other regions of the spine are similarly identified. See Figure 2.)

The sacrum is a solid, triangular-shaped bone that is attached to the two sides of the pelvis. Although it is solid, it is formed by the fusion of five separate bones into one. The famous sacroiliac joint is the juncture on the side of the sacrum and the iliac bone of the pelvis. (See Figures 1 and 2.) In the past, this joint had been unjustly accused of being the source of a large percentage of back problems. In fact, forty to fifty years ago, fusion of this joint was a popular procedure for relief of back pain. We now know that although it feels as though the pain emanates from the sacroiliac joint, it is usually referred from somewhere else. Fusion of the sacroiliac joint is rarely performed these days.

One more bony landmark is of importance, the little vestigial tailbone known as the *coccyx*. If you have ever fallen in a sitting position, you already know where that bone is located. It can easily be felt at the very lower tip of the sacrum as a small hornlike projection that bends inward. Bumping on your bottom can bruise or even break the small bone, causing considerable pain for several weeks. After delivery of a baby, many women are acutely aware of tenderness in the coccyx when they sit or get up from a chair.

About 20 percent of all people have some variation in the form and structure of the vertebral body. Occasionally a vertebral body is only half-formed. Sometimes people may only have four lumbar vertebrae, and others may have six. The sacrum may not be a solid bone, but instead the upper segments may be slightly separated. Occasionally the back of the spinal column remains open so that the normal protective shell is partially absent. These things do occur, but for the most part these abnormalities do not cause pain. However, they are some of the things that doctors look for when they examine X-rays.

Ligaments

Ligaments are the tough, strong bands of tissue that connect bones. (See Figure 4.) All you skiers know about the ligaments in your knees and how wobbly and unstable the knee becomes when those connecting ligaments are torn. Well, the ligaments in your back can get torn as well. Fortunately, because of the complex structure of the connections between the bones, when this happens, the joint does not become wobbly like a knee but has some mild instability that can lead to pain and discomfort. There are two major ligaments in the spine, which strap all the vertebral bones together. The one in front of the vertebral bones is the anterior longitudinal ligament, and the one behind but in front of the spinal cord is the posterior longitudinal ligament. These ligaments limit movement between

LIGAMENTS #4

FROM BEHIND

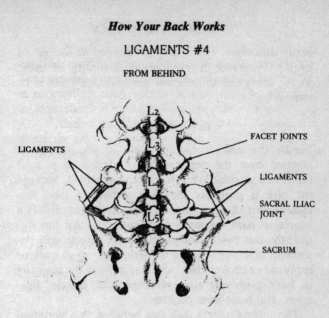

LIGAMENTS

FACET JOINTS

LIGAMENTS

SACRAL ILIAC JOINT

SACRUM

L2
L3
L4
L5

the vertebral bones and also help keep the intervertebral disk in place. Multiple small ligaments provide attachment for other portions of the vertebral bodies.

The Facet Joints

I have already alluded to these joints. They are small joints on the back of the vertebral bodies, which limit movement between the bones. (See Figures 2 and 4.) Excessive sudden jolting in any direction, especially a twisting type of movement, can irritate and inflame them. Characteristically when they are inflamed, you are literally "bent out of shape" or twisted to the side. Manipulating the back may bring about relief from pain and spasm. Often it is described as "something slipping back into place." Actually the facet joint never really dislocates, but it may get hinged or locked on itself. Gymnasts develop great flexibility in these joints; otherwise those great acrobatic feats would be impossible.

Intervertebral Disk

Finally the disk! I suspect some of you may have skipped over the previous parts of this chapter to reach this section. Well, it is not unexpected, because the disk is probably the most publicized (and maligned) part of your spine. Undoubtedly the disk is a source of pain for many back sufferers. All too frequently, however, back problems are erroneously described as being due to a herniated or slipped or ruptured or broken disk, whereas in truth the majority of back problems are associated with muscle, ligament, and facet-joint problems.

The intervertebral disk lies between two vertebral bodies. On the surface of each of the bodies is a thin, slatelike structure composed of a gritty cartilage substance. These *end plates* protect the body of each vertebra. On the outside or periphery of the vertebral bodies is a thick ligament that connects the edges of the two vertebral bodies together. This is the *annulus fibrosis,* and not only does it connect the vertebral bodies, but it also holds inside, between the two vertebral bodies, the part that everyone refers to as the *disk*. (See Figure 5).

This "disk," anatomically known as the *nucleus pulposus,* occupies the center portion of the space and represents only about one third of the entire structure. It is a firm, gelatinlike substance that can be compressed in any direction, and like a cushion can absorb tremendous pressure and deformation without breaking. When the pressure is removed, it can restore itself

DISK (ANNULUS FIBROSIS) #5

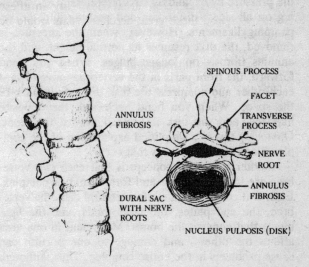

SPINOUS PROCESS

FACET

TRANSVERSE PROCESS

ANNULUS FIBROSIS

NERVE ROOT

ANNULUS FIBROSIS

DURAL SAC WITH NERVE ROOTS

NUCLEUS PULPOSIS (DISK)

to its normal dimensions. This dramatic ability is the result of a high water content. If you fill a balloon with water, it can adjust to any shape you choose, and although the shape changes, the volume of water never changes. Have you ever slept on a water mattress? Well, for some it can be quite comfortable, and although the mattress is turgid when filled with water, there is still enough flexibility so that each contour of your body is gently molded into the mattress. When you arise, the mattress is flat again. (However, for many of my patients, sleeping on a water bed is uncomfortable.)

The center portion of the disk is confined in a limited space by the end plates of the vertebrae and by the surrounding tough and durable annulus fibrosis. Standing, bending, running, jumping, and lifting compress this disk inside the space, and the disk reacts to the pressure by expanding circumferentially and pressing on all sides, distending and pushing into the restraining ligaments. However, when the pressure is removed, the disk resumes its normal height, and the annulus fibrosis no longer bulges. When you bend forward, the front parts of the vertebrae move toward each other and compress the disk toward the back of the space. When you bend backward, the opposite happens, and the disk is pressed toward the front. Obviously this is a simplified explanation of the complex biomechanical events that occur.

Another important concept is that each two vertebrae are linked together and form a unit or complex. Each unit consists of the intervertebral disk, the vertebrae, the end plates, the facet joints, and the ligaments that connect the bones. Movement in one area affects the others, and damage to one portion can cause problems in the entire complex. Thus, although a back problem may be accredited to a facet injury or to a slipped disk or to a torn ligament, the entire complex or unit is involved, and eventual restoration to normal function requires attention to all of these parts.

Let us return to the disk again (remember, I am referring to the central gelatinous portion). As noted, most of its wonderful properties are attributable to its water content (85 percent). The bad news is that as one ages, the water content diminishes. This process begins in the late twenties and by age forty the water content of the disk is down to 70 percent. That means that the disk has less ability to withstand pressure and to resume its normal height. Speaking of height, those of you under age forty might have noted that if you measure yourself in the morning, you may be one inch taller than if you measure yourself at night. The constant compression of the disk in the upright or sitting position pushes some of the water out of the disk. At night when you are lying in bed and recumbent and the compression is removed, the water is absorbed back into the disk, causing it to expand. Although the expansion of each disk is minuscule, when each tiny addition is multiplied by the number of disks, the overall height increase can be significant. It was a common phenomenon for astronauts returning from an extended time in space, where there is no gravity to compress the disks, to be two inches taller than when they left. However, after a short time back on earth, they returned to their normal height.

A slipped, herniated, or ruptured disk means that the annulus fibrosis has given way to the inner pressures and allowed a portion or all of the nucleus pulposus to protrude, usually backward and to the side. When this occurs, the nerve root that lies against the disk space can be compressed by a protrusion of the disk. This compression is not only painful, but can cause significant neurological problems. More about that later.

If all disks lose their water content as one ages, then why doesn't everyone have a back problem? Certainly everyone has the potential for back problems, and you might even say that no one will go unscathed. In fact, do you know of an adult who has never complained of a backache? Which is not to imply that everyone has a serious problem. Some people have inherently stronger disks than others, some have been fortunate in avoiding damaging stress to the back, and others have developed strong muscles that protect the back. Even these people, however, should be alert to aches and twinges that may portend a future serious back problem.

The Nerves

The billions of cells that comprise the brain are connected to the body by nerves that bring information from our environment to the brain to process and then send instructions to various muscles for an appropriate response to that information. This instantaneous system is made possible by our sensory organs (the eyes, ears, nose, mouth) and by the spinal cord with its nerve roots, which supply the nerves that provide sensation to our hands and feet, and also the nerves that cause our muscles to function.

At each intervertebral level a nerve root branches off the spinal cord and exits the spinal column to a final destination, such as a particular muscle, bone, joint, or area of skin. Each nerve root is numbered according to the level at which it exits. As an example, the L4 nerve root emerges between the L4 and L5 vertebrae, and the L5 nerve root between the L5–S1 vertebrae (Figure 6). When a disk herniates, it compresses the nerve root that crosses behind the interspace. Thus a disk herniation involving the L4–5 disk would compress the L5 nerve root as it passes down to exit beneath the pedicle of L5, and a disk herniation at L5–S1 would entrap the S1 nerve root as it passes below the pedicle of S1. As I mentioned, 95 percent of all disk herniations occur at L4–L5 and L5–S1 levels. If the disk herniation occurs at L4–L5, the L5 nerve root is compressed. If the herniation occurs at L5–S1, the S1 nerve root is involved. Occasionally there is a variation in the way a nerve departs from the spinal canal, or a disk protrusion can be so large that two nerves are compromised. Although rare, these abnormalities can cause difficulty in diagnosis and treatment of disk and nerve problems.

In the infant, the spinal cord extends from the skull

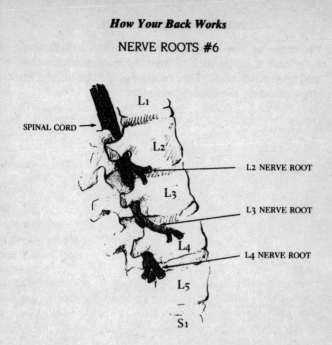

to the lowest part of the spine, but as the child grows, the spinal cord becomes relatively shorter, so that in an adult the cord itself extends only to the L1 level. However, the nerve roots continue in the dural sac, which extends into the sacrum, and exit at the appropriate levels. Thus, the lower part of the dural sac contains only the nerve roots, and not the spinal cord itself. Because the spinal cord does not descend to the lumbar region, many interspinal procedures can be safely performed in the lower portion of the back, such as spinal taps, myelograms, and epidural and spinal anesthesia.

Your anatomy lesson is over. I trust that it has not been too technical, but don't worry if you forget some of the terms. Periodically I will repeat explanations of the terms as they occur. More relevantly, I think you now have a better idea of how the back is structured and how it functions. This knowledge will be helpful in understanding the ensuing chapters.

3. What Can Go Wrong with Your Back

THE SYMPTOMS OF BACK PROBLEMS

If you have never experienced back problems, this next section may seem superfluous. However, if you have had back pain or the spasm and stiffness that are associated with it, or the agonizing shooting sciatic pain in your legs, the following descriptions may be all too familiar. What I shall do is describe the various types of pain you may have and then relate those pains to specific disorders and problems. I shall then discuss these underlying disorders in greater detail. I shall point out the significance of the pain, where it is, its relationship to duration, and the effect of body posture upon it.

One of the most difficult aspects of analyzing someone's back pain is to determine what the person means by pain in the lower back. Three different symptoms are associated with the "low-back syndrome." The first is typically pain in the lower back and occasionally in the upper-buttock area. Second is pain that radiates into the thigh and leg, often as far down as the ankle and foot. This latter pain is known as *sciatica*. The third type is cramping sensations in the thigh and calves usually associated with standing and walking.

Low-Back Pain

Typical low-back pain, or *lumbago* as it was once called, is related to a mechanical problem in the lower back and is not usually associated with a ruptured disk or pinched nerve. It can be caused by inflammation of the facet joint, strain of the supporting muscles, arthritis, or local conditions that can cause stress on the supporting structures or bones. Our understanding of the actual mechanism of pain in the lower back is still far from complete, but we do know that small nerves supply the ligaments, muscles, and bones in the area, and any injury or inflammation of these nerves can produce local pain. Muscle spasm, which is painful, sustained contraction of muscles, is often associated with low-back pain. Whether the muscle spasm is the cause or result of pain is still controversial. Much research has been done to determine if pain emanating from the underlying disk, ligaments, or bones causes the muscle spasm, or whether the muscle is "injured" and then goes into spasm. I believe that in most cases the problem starts with the underlying structures and involves the muscles secondarily. However, there are instances where the muscles can actually be directly injured or strained and thus are primarily responsible for pain. As far as you the patient are concerned, your back hurts regardless of the source.

Leg Pain (Sciatic Pain)

The sciatic nerve, which is the main nerve in the leg, is also the largest nerve in the body. Irritation of this nerve can produce pain that starts in the lower-back or buttock area and radiates all the way down the back of the leg to the foot and toes. Classically this pain is caused by compression of a nerve root due to herniation or rupture of an intervertebral disk. Five different nerve roots from the lower-lumbar and upper-sacral regions combine to form the sciatic nerve. A disk protrusion in any of these areas could result in pain along the course of the nerve. Sciatic pain can be present with or without low-back pain. Herniation of a disk with compression of a nerve at a higher level, such as L2–L3 or L3–L4, may produce pain in the front of the thigh. This type of pain is known as *femoral neuritis* because the nerve roots to the femoral nerve are involved.

Cramping or Heaviness in the Legs
(Pseudoclaudication)

The third type of pain related to the lower-back syndrome involves cramping or heaviness in the legs associated with prolonged standing and walking. This pain rapidly subsides with sitting or rest. It is due to spinal stenosis or narrowing of the spinal canal and the *foramen* (a small passageway through which the nerve roots exit). People who have this condition find that if they lean forward while walking, they are able to walk longer distances before the pain begins. This cramping type of pain is to be differentiated from the cramps that people develop in their legs due to circulatory insufficiency, which is known as *intermittent claudication*. Most people with circulatory insufficiency will have pain only with walking, while people with *pseudoclaudication* (associated with spinal stenosis) will have pain standing as well. Weakness in the legs, pins and needles in the feet, or numbness of the soles of the feet are also associated with the syndrome of spinal stenosis.

Generally back pain is only vaguely described by the patient. To help patients better explain their symptoms, I often provide them with a list of adjectives that describe the pain in various ways and also with a diagram of a person, both front and back, so that they pinpoint the location of the pain. Only with careful questioning can a doctor discover that the pain may be localized to the lower back, spread across the area, or may be predominantly on one side or the other. The major focus of the pain may be in the buttock area. The pain itself may radiate or spread down the leg, either into the thigh or all the way down to the foot. It may spread around the pelvic area to the front of the abdomen, or occasionally it may radiate into the mid- or upper-back area between the shoulder blades. It may be a dull nagging ache that comes and goes and is usually worse with fatigue and at the end of the day. Tension and stress can certainly make it worse. The pain can be dull, minor, intermittent, and not disabling. It can be severe, lacerating, or knifelike, resulting in agony that makes it impossible to move. Patients have often told me of literally crawling to the bathroom on their hands and knees because the pain was too severe for them to stand. When the pain is that bad, you become completely immobilized and are unable to change positions without experiencing several moments of agony.

If the pain radiates down the leg to below the knee, it is usually the result of pressure on the sciatic nerve. That type of leg pain is called, as you might expect, *sciatica*. As noted, sciatica is often caused by the disk protruding backward and causing pressure or pinching of the adjacent nerve roots.

Some pain may be present only in the morning when you first get out of bed. You experience a sense of soreness and stiffness in the lower back that eases after a hot shower and after you have been walking about for a while. This is typical of arthritic pain.

Other pains may occur only with standing and walking but are relieved by sitting and lying down. A sense of heaviness in the thighs may accompany these symptoms. After walking for a few blocks, your leg pain may become so intense that you have to stop and rest, allowing the pain to subside before you can resume walking. Older people often complain of these symptoms, which may be related to a narrowing of the vertebral canal in the lower back. This narrowing, which is known as *spinal stenosis,* squeezes the nerve roots and causes pain.

A perplexing problem is the pain that is felt in the back without the back being the culprit. Patients with kidney stones or other types of kidney problems may experience back pain. The same symptom can occur with prostate problems, uterus problems, or even with infections or inflammation of the lungs. This pain is known as *referred pain,* because the site of the problem is not where the pain is perceived. Heart attacks often produce pain radiating into the left arm. Gallbladder pain is frequently experienced as pain in the right shoulder. Careful analysis of the pain symptoms and a thorough physical examination can differentiate referred pain from true back problems. For instance, whereas most people with low-back pain can get comfortable lying in bed, patients with pain from an inflamed or infected kidney generally feel better sitting or standing. These little clues are important in determining the origin of the pain.

BAD POSTURE, A MAJOR CAUSE OF BACK PAIN

From the ballet room to the military parade ground, posture is constantly stressed. Utterance of this word brings to mind someone trying to stand "straight" (head up, shoulder back, stomach in), or a model walking with a book on her head, or the Third World native carrying a bundle of wood or a bowl upon his or her head. Yes, posture refers to all of these, but to much more as well. I would like to define posture as the position of your body in space, whether it be standing, sitting, or lying down. In every instance, it is your "back" that determines the attitude of your body.

Your spine literally supports your upper body. It is constantly being strained while standing, sitting, bending, twisting, and lifting. The only time it rests and the stresses are relieved is when you are lying down.

Even then, however, if you lie down improperly, your back may not obtain the rest it needs. After a while, the unrested back is not able to perform its work, and that is when the trouble begins. You would not think of running a marathon without training. Then why put your back through the "marathon of life" without proper training and strengthening? Indeed, that is what this book is about—learning how to prepare your back for the run through life. I say *run* purposely, because in our modern world, we never seem to have time to walk. We are always running, rushing, under great tension and stress, not getting adequate rest or sleep, and paying little attention to the general condition of our bodies, let alone our backs.

Good posture helps to relieve the strain on your back. It distributes the forces that act upon your spine over a greater area, thus dissipating the pressures on specific regions. Good posture allows your muscles to relax in between moments of work. Smooth movements put less stress on the muscles than awkward and sudden movements. Let us consider posture and all its major components.

I have described the construction of the spine, and now is the time to visualize the sum of the parts. When you stand up, your back from the base of the skull to the pelvis assumes a certain configuration. When viewed from behind, the spine is straight. A line drawn on the spine from the base of the skull to the floor would descend without lateral (sideways) deviation in most people.

However, occasionally the spine deviates to one side or may deviate to one side in the upper-dorsal area and to the opposite side in the lower-lumbar region. (See Figure 7.) This deviation or curve is known as *scoliosis*. It occurs mostly in young teenage girls as the result of growth abnormalities of which we are still ignorant. In rare instances, congenital malformation of the bone or muscular paralysis cause scoliosis. Severe curves with lateral displacement can be treated with braces and/or surgery. Scoliosis can be diagnosed in most cases by looking at a person's back when she or he stands up and bends over. X-rays are necessary to determine the actual degree of the curve. Treatment of scoliosis will be discussed in the chapter on back problems of children.

On the other hand, if we look at the normal spine from the side, we note immediately that the spine is not straight. The cervical spine bends forward *(lordosis)*, the dorsal spine bends backward *(kyphosis)*, the lumbar spine bends forward, and the sacrum bends backward. It is readily apparent that each curve is opposite to the one above, and the magnitude of each curve is about the same. This is normal. The curves act to distribute the forces of weight bearing, lifting, and bending over the entire torso. They provide strength and mobility for the necessary movements of the spine.

These curves may become exaggerated—the cervical lordosis is markedly increased, the dorsal kyphosis becomes prominent, the shoulders get rounded, and the lumbar spine compensates by developing a severe swayback posture, causing the sacrum to stick out and

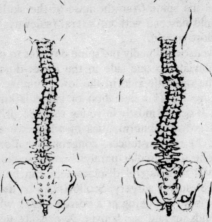

SINGLE CURVE IN
DORSAL SPINE

DOUBLE CURVE IN
DORSAL & LUMBAR

become almost horizontal. Instead of supporting and facilitating spinal mobility, these exaggerated curves produce intensely aggravated stress throughout the spine, especially in the lower lumbar region. The excessive stress produced by the exaggerated curves eventually wears down the joints, disks, muscles, and ligaments that support the spine, resulting in pain, stiffness, and considerable discomfort.

You might ask whether a perfectly straight spine is desirable; surprisingly the answer is no! If the spine is straight, then something is wrong. Remember, those gentle curves facilitate movement and protect the spine in all its functions. Someone who has muscle spasms as a result of a cervical strain or injury will have straightening of the neck and loss of the normal cervical lordosis until the muscle spasms subside. This dra-

BAD POSTURE #8

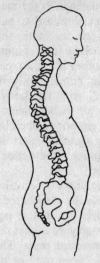

matic straightening of the cervical spine is readily seen on physical examination and an X-ray of the neck. Similarly, normal lumbar lordosis is lost when the lower-back muscles are in spasm.

In summary, posture is the relationship of the various structural parts of the body to each other: the head, the spine, and the pelvis are the major components. Good posture implies that this relationship is in a proper or healthful alignment. Poor posture means that this relationship is distorted, and abnormal strains on the spine are being produced as the result of this malalignment.

Engineers are well aware of the damage that malalignment (or imbalance) can cause to machines. Your automatic washer is a case in point. If the clothes in the tub are not balanced during the spin cycle, the tub will rotate in an erratic, violent motion, which can cause considerable damage to the machine by eroding or wearing out crucial movable parts. In order to avoid this damage, an automatic shutoff is installed that prevents the machine from spinning at high speeds when the load of clothes is unbalanced.

Unfortunately the human body does not have a mechanism that will stop the body from operating when an imbalance (or malalignment) is present. The body does, however, respond (albeit belatedly) by emitting painful warning signals to alert the body occupant that something is amiss. Woe betide the person who ignores these signals!

With poor posture and excessive lordosis or kyphosis, pressure is unequally distributed along the vertebral bodies and disks so that a portion wears out prematurely. Regrettably we cannot replace spinal parts as we can washing-machine parts. Therefore, once an area of our back is "worn out" or damaged, we just have to keep using it. Good posture delays that tendency for early wearing or degeneration. Good posture helps to maintain proper back alignment and to preserve good healthy-back mechanics, and although it may not entirely prevent wearing out of the structures, it certainly delays the process and ensures a healthier back for many more years.

But what if the horse has already left the barn? If the wearing is already present? Is all lost? Should you just give up and confine yourself to a rocking chair? By no means. You can help yourself; in most instances, you can improve your posture, remove that abnormal stress on the weakened areas, adjust the load, and continue to lead an active and full life. But it does require persistent effort on your part to think constantly about your posture and keep doing exercises for your back every day. It is not easy, but it can be done. In the latter part of this book, I shall tell you how.

The message is that good posture prevents problems, and poor posture results in pain. In fact, I strongly believe, along with many other experts who treat back problems, that the great majority of back pains are related to poor posture. All of us know people who slouch when standing and yet do not have back pain. Does that disprove this theory? No, because the results of poor posture are cumulative. That is, over a period of time, the abnormal stresses gradually wear down the involved structures until eventually the dike gives way and the water rushes through. It is not tying your shoelace, opening a stuck window, or a sudden sneeze that throws your back out and causes pain. Rather, it is the long, constant misuse of the back that has slowly, progressively worn away the support and weakened the muscles that ultimately leads to that painful and sometimes agonizing moment of "back pain." Be wise, take care of your back before you have trouble. Improve your posture and strengthen the muscles that support and protect your spine.

Up to now, I have emphasized poor posture as a major underlying cause of back pain and discomfort. Now, I shall discuss in detail pain and symptoms associated with specific problems. I shall describe disk pain, arthritic pain, acute injuries to the back, conditions that cause instability of the back, problems associated with the aging process, referred pain, and finally the relationship of stress and tension to lower-back problems.

NO MORE ACHING BACK

INTERVERTEBRAL DISK

I shall begin this discussion with the slipped disk, because it is often cited (mistakenly) as the major cause of back problems. Ever since Mixter and Barr, a neurosurgeon and an orthopedic surgeon in Boston, wrote their paper on the relief of back and sciatic pain by removing a herniated disk, the world has come to know about the association of disk herniation and back and leg pain. These two men published their paper in 1934 in *The New England Journal of Medicine*, but before that, disk degeneration and herniation had been described by Schmorl in his excellent monograph on the pathological anatomy of the spine that was published in Germany in 1932. However, the connection between disk herniation, back pain, and sciatica was proven by Mixter and Barr. Their study demonstrated that after removal of a herniated disk, the symptoms of pains in the back and leg were relieved.

In the half-century that has passed since the publication of that paper, the slipped disk has grown from an obscure cause of pain to the predominant cause of back problems, at least in the minds of the general public. Ninety percent of the patients whom I see for back pain tell me at the onset, "I have a slipped disk." Sometimes they have actually been examined and properly diagnosed by a physician. Other times they have pain and assume the problem is a slipped or ruptured disk. At any rate, contrary to common belief, disk herniations are not the predominant cause of low-back pain. (The most common cause is poor posture and constant stress or strain on the structures of the lower back, the ligaments, joints, and muscles.) Occasionally some individuals have naturally weaker or less structurally sound intervertebral disks. These people tend to have disk problems at several levels rather than just at the two lower levels in which most disk herniations occur (L5–S1 and L4–L5). Also, these same individuals generally have a more extensive family history of back and disk problems.

In most instances, disk herniation is a late sequel to chronic back stress. The individual segments have been weakened over a period of time, and when the muscles are particularly fatigued, an unsound mechanical maneuver, such as a sudden twist or lifting without protecting the back, forces the disk against the weakened annulus fibrosis. At first it bulges outward. If the force is sufficient or is maintained over a long period of time, the disk eventually pokes through the ligament and protrudes into the spinal canal. Under extreme pressure, it occasionally ruptures out with such force that the entire fragment lies free within the canal or in the nerve-root foramen. This bulging or protruding disk presses on the spinal nerve root, and pain radiates down the leg. (See Figure 9.) The pain typically travels along the course of the sciatic nerve, which runs through the buttock, thigh, leg, and foot.

One of the most confusing things about disk problems is the terminology. I have just described the sequence of events when the disk pushes against and then through the restraining ligament (the annulus fibrosis). While I can almost always determine if the disk is part or most of the problem by history and physical examination, I usually cannot differentiate whether the disk is bulging, protruding, or completely extruded. (See Figure 10.) The severity of symptoms and degree of nerve involvement—weakness, loss of reflexes, numbness or atrophy—only suggest the extent of disk herniation.

Special tests and procedures that I discuss in the next chapter are necessary to determine the degree of disk herniation. Standard X-rays only show the bone

DISK PRESSING ON NERVE #9

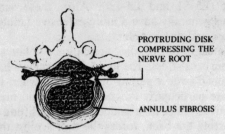

PROTRUDING DISK
COMPRESSING THE
NERVE ROOT

ANNULUS FIBROSIS

structure and are not helpful in determining disk herniation. The CAT scan (computerized axial tomography), the MRI (magnetic resonance imaging) and a myelogram are helpful in visualizing the degree of disk protrusion. However, these are all procedures that are done later in the course of events and not on initial examination except in unusual circumstances. If I suspect that the disk is damaged, I may describe the condition to my patient as a "slipped disk," "bulging disk," "protruding disk," or "herniated disk." I may even say the disk is ruptured. These terms all refer to the fact that the nucleus pulposus or soft central portion of the disk no longer occupies its central location and has been forced backward, pushing the restraining ligament outward or even tearing through it.

It is important to remember that once the disk is herniated, it never returns to its former place. When the nucleus pulposus is forced from the center of the disk space, the segmental complex between the two vertebral bodies is altered, and the space narrows *forever*. Even a partially herniated disk will result in some narrowing of the disk space. This narrowing, which may become evident on X-ray, places stress on the facet joints that are impinging upon each other. Because of this impingement, the nerve-root canal is

DEGREE OF HERNIATION #10

BULGING DISK   PROTRUDING DISK   EXTRUDED DISK

also narrowed, and as time goes by, arthritic spurs along the facet joints further narrow the canal. Finally the protruding disk itself can press upon the adjacent nerve root, pinching it, compressing it, or in some cases even crushing it.

Any pressure on the nerve root causes an electrical impulse to pass along its length, and that impulse is what we perceive as pain. As I said before, depending upon which nerve root is involved, the pain can radiate down the back of the leg to the heel, the big toe, or the little toe. Occasionally the pain may radiate into the buttock or into the front of the thigh. These pains are all manifestations of pressure on a nerve root.

Now, you might ask again, if the disk is protruding and pressing on the nerve, and the disk never goes back into place, how can you eliminate the pain? The answer lies in the anatomy of the spinal canal. In most normal-sized canals, the space is large enough for the protruding disk and the nerve root to coexist peacefully. Picture in your mind the ruptured disk pushing against the nerve, which is bent over the bulging portion. (See Figure 9.) If the canal is large enough, the nerve is simply lifted away from the edge of the bone. Initially, when the disk first extrudes and strikes against the nerve, there is significant pain, but when the nerve inflammation subsides, as long as the nerve is not being compressed against the bone in the canal, the pain goes away. However, if the canal is narrow and the disk compresses the nerve against the canal wall, the pain will persist until the pressure is somehow removed. In order to illustrate what can happen, I shall describe the case history of two of my back patients.

First, Mr. R. is a forty-one-year-old Wall Street investment banker who works sixteen hours a day and spends his weekends on the phone at his desk. He believes in exercise, but just never has the time for it. His back and stomach are in fair-to-poor shape. His posture is satisfactory, but as the day progresses, it worsens. He slouches when standing and sitting. Even in bed, he tosses and turns, his back sagging in the soft mattress his wife loves. He has ignored periodic episodes of low-back pain and stiffness in spite of the fact that there have been times he was bent over with spasms. Additionally he has had twinges of pain in his right leg. Nevertheless, he would just "tough it out," and eventually his back would return to "normal."

If we could look into his spine, we would find that during these past several years, the disk was gradually pushing against and distorting the annulus fibrosis. This localized weakness and thinning of the ligament allowed the nucleus pulposus (the portion we commonly refer to as the "disk") to bulge into the spinal canal. However, it never actually ruptured through the ligament. The intervertebral disk space was gradually becoming narrower as the disk was wearing down due to the constant pressure. The facet joints had been increasingly stressed and strained because with the narrowing of the disk space they were pushed together. The muscles that support the entire complex were weakened and just barely able to do their job, especially at the end of a fourteen- or sixteen-hour workday. Every so often, the muscles were not able to sustain the effort, and the disk would push out a little further, irritating the adjacent nerve and causing a spasm. Additionally the facet joints were being continually rubbed "the wrong way."

That's what was happening in Mr. R.'s back. Those spasms in his back represented the pain derived from the inability of the weak muscles and facet joints to do their jobs properly. The pain in his leg resulted from nerve irritation caused by the bulging disk. Rest eliminated the spasms, and gradually he got relief from the pain. But Mr. R. was walking a thin line.

One day after driving home from work, he twisted around in the front seat to pick up his briefcase from the backseat of the car. As he lifted it up, he experienced an excruciating pain in his lower back, radiating into his buttocks and down the back of the right leg and foot. He described it as "like being stabbed by a hot knife." For a moment, he could barely breathe, and then, with the utmost caution, he slid himself out of the car. He could not straighten up, and was bent over to the side. Each step he took was agony, and finally he dropped to the ground, crawled to his house on his hands and knees, and collapsed on the floor in front of his wife. What happened in his case was that the disk had been forced through the ligament and smashed right against the adjacent nerve root—like a sledgehammer pulverizing a rock. *OUCH!*

Mrs. R. helped him to bed, rushed for whatever pain medication they had in the house, and called frantically for a doctor. Bed rest and further medication were recommended. After several days, the awful pain eased. Mr. R. was able to get out of bed, albeit with some discomfort. After three weeks, he was well enough to return to work. However, he continued to have some aches and discomfort for an additional three months.

Let's look again into Mr. R.'s back. Lucky for him

the canal was wide enough so that even though the protruding disk was pushing against the nerve root, that structure had accommodated to the pressure and was not compressed against the bony wall. In addition, the initial swelling of the nerve root caused by the rupture of the disk disappeared. The torn ligaments were healing, the fragment of disk was contracting, and the facet-joint inflammation had subsided. Although the pain had dissipated, the damage had been done and would remain forever. Mr. R.'s back will always be vulnerable to further attacks, some of which may be even more severe. If he had paid heed to the initial warning signs and improved his posture, begun an exercise program for his back, and worked on stress-reduction activities (such as athletics and general exercises), he might have avoided this terrible scenario. However, though he is in trouble, it's not too late to begin a rehabilitation program of exercises and life-style modification.

The other case history I shall present concerns Mrs. B., a woman in her middle thirties who prides herself on being "in shape." She leads a full life. She is married, has two children, ages four and six, and does free-lance writing. For years, she had attended aerobics class three times weekly, and although she did not have a fetish about her diet, she carefully kept her weight at an appropriate level for her height and body build.

Over the past two years, she had to cope with many serious problems in her life. Her mother was ill for many months. Her husband had to change his job, and they moved to a new city. Both their incomes were reduced. She had no help with her children. Her older child was in first grade, but her younger child was still at home. She had stopped aerobics classes because they had become too expensive for her, and she just didn't have the time or the discipline to do them at home by herself. She spent more time at her typewriter trying to earn additional money for the family. The household chores persisted, and every time she turned around, someone was making demands upon her time and energy. However, she felt she was coping pretty well in spite of everything. She didn't scold her children excessively, she could listen patiently to her husband's worries and concerns, and she was able to console her parents regarding their health problems. She had the determination to rewrite that story once again so it would really be perfect, and she could accept with minimal remorse another rejection by her editor. So what if she had a constant ache in her back, if she had difficulty lifting the little one off the floor, or if vacuuming the rug was a chore she detested? She could live with that—no problem, or so she thought.

On her and her husband's last vacation together, the first four days on the Caribbean island had been glorious. Just the two of them, alone again like honeymooners, basking in the sun, without the daily pressures of home. Surely a sore back after one set of singles tennis was normal for someone who was "out of shape." Nothing that a couple of aspirin and a hot shower could not cure. Anyway, by the time dinner was over and an adequate amount of red wine consumed, she felt no pain at all. Then, back in their room alone, feeling amorous, adventurous, and enthusiastic, she found making love utterly wonderful.

Suddenly she felt something literally "snap" in her back, followed by a momentary numbness in her entire left leg and then a severe pain in her left buttock that seared down the back of her left leg to her foot. She screamed with pain. Her concerned husband thought at first that he had hurt her. She gaspingly described the pain to him. The hotel doctor was called.

He examined her and found that the muscles in her left foot were weak. She had no ankle reflex, and the side of her left foot was numb. "You have a herniated disk," he said. "Your nerve is being paralyzed, and you had better get to a hospital right away."

Now, let us look at the case closely. This young, vigorous woman had formerly always taken care of herself, but for the past two years had not exercised, and had been too involved with her family and her work to think about her back. She had always been healthy, and had never had a serious illness or even surgery. The only time she had been in the hospital was to give birth to her two children, and she had breezed through both labors and deliveries. She used to laugh at her father with his back. He was always going to a chiropractor, wearing a brace, having acupuncture, or taking some new medication. It had been easy for her to tease him that he was just "getting old." After all, her young back had always been healthy. What happened?

What happened was that even though her posture was fair, she put more stress on her back than the muscles could tolerate. The disks had a hereditary tendency to wear out early, inherited from her father. The annulus fibrosis was constantly being stretched and weakened. Those early signs of an aching back were ignored. Then, while making love, she hyperextended and flexed her lower back with such force that the disk ruptured through the annulus and compressed the nerve against the bony canal, causing pain and muscle weakness. There was no room for the nerve to escape from the pressure, and it was impossible for the disk to go back into the intervertebral space.

By the time the patient returned from her trip and arrived at the hospital where I examined her, the symptoms were worse. The numbness and weakness had become more severe. The sciatic pain was somewhat less, but she could not lie flat on her back. She had to have several pillows underneath her knees or lie on her side with her knees and hips flexed (fetal position). Coughing or sneezing would cause excruciating pain down the left leg. Even when she tried to laugh, it hurt. An emergency myelogram was performed. This confirmed my clinical impression that she had a completely extruded disk pressing on the nerve. Bed rest and medication would never cure that situation. The next day, I operated and removed the disk. When the patient awoke from anesthesia, the leg pain had gone. She was home within one week. She began exercises in three weeks. She was almost back to normal by three months. Eventually she regained normal sensation and muscle strength in her left leg.

The moral of these two case histories is that not all disk herniations are the same or can be treated in the same fashion. Anatomical variation in the size of the canal, the magnitude of the herniation, the position of the nerves, and the health of the muscles are all important to how well the patient does. Be of good cheer, however, because although 80 million Americans suffer from back problems, and a large number of these have disk trouble, 90 percent of all patients get better within two months, and 60 percent get better within three weeks. So the odds are in your favor. The 90 percent of the people who get better in two months do so almost regardless of what kind of treatment is provided. Therefore, relief is mainly a matter of time, helped by rest, medication, and avoidance of strain. Mr. R. got better without surgery. Mrs. B. required an operation to remove the disk in order to get better. Mr. R. had enough space for the slipped disk and nerve root to coexist. Mrs. B. did not, so surgery was required.

I wish to emphasize at this time that it is not always so easy to recognize which disk problems require surgery and which ones should be treated conservatively. Basically all slipped disks should be treated conservatively with nonsurgical procedures. Surgery is indicated for those relatively few patients who have paralysis or weakness of the muscles associated with disk herniation, or who have severe or persistent pain that interferes with their functional activities and is not relieved by the usual conservative means.

Most disk herniations occur in persons between thirty-five to fifty years of age. These are the years when people are still very physically active and usually not getting enough rest, while simultaneously their disks are losing water and becoming more vulnerable.

Heredity, work patterns, posture, stress, and lack of exercise all play an important role in the development of disk problems.

Let us return to our two patients. One year after their recoveries, Mr. R. and Mrs. B. are leading full, active lives. They are slowly slipping back into their old patterns of too little rest, too much stress, and not enough exercise. So far, they have no pain and believe they are really "cured." Unfortunately they're wrong. Surgically removing the disk or relieving the pain with bed rest does not cure the underlying lack of mechanical stability. That segmental complex of the intervertebral disk, facet joint, and adjacent vertebral bodies will never be the same again. The mechanics are altered forever. They will never function exactly as they did before the injuries occurred. Precisely because they will never be the same, it is essential for Mr. R. and Mrs. B. to protect their weakened areas by strengthening the supporting muscles through back exercises and good posture.

Although the two patients I have described are both

active individuals and under stress, I have numerous patients who are sedentary, never exercise, and never seem to stress themselves, and yet they too have developed back and disk problems.

Unless you protect weak areas by exercising daily, you are almost certain to have a recurrence of symptoms, either at the same disk or an adjacent one. Remember, you never cure a back problem, you only control it, and that control is achieved by good body mechanics, good posture, and regular exercises that maintain strong muscles.

SPINAL STENOSIS

As I mentioned earlier, lumbar-spine stenosis is a narrowing of the spinal canal in the lumbar area that can squeeze the nerve roots and cause low-back pain, sciatic-type pain, pseudoclaudication (cramping in the legs), or all three. The narrowing (stenosis) is generally the result of a buildup of arthritis and degenerating bulging disks. These can occur at one level or at several levels. That is, the narrowing can occur just at the L4–L5 level, or it may extend from the L1 level to the sacrum. People with longstanding spondylolysis or spondylolisthesis (more about these later) are prone to develop localized areas of narrowing with the typical symptoms of stenosis. Occasionally the canal itself is congenitally smaller than normal, and in these instances, the involved individuals are predisposed to develop this condition. Spinal stenosis generally occurs in people over sixty years of age. The symptoms may be very vague in the beginning, starting with low-back pain, a heavy feeling in the back of the thighs when walking, and, finally, cramping pain in the legs after walking just one or two blocks. The pain is relieved by sitting down or resting. The relief is almost immediate. Knee and ankle reflexes may be diminished or absent. Sensation is usually intact, although occasionally vibratory sensation may be diminished. Patients often complain of numbness in their feet, but when tested, sensation is normal. The ability to straight-leg raise is not impaired. Muscle strength is preserved until the stenosis is far advanced. Although the clinical findings are not very dramatic, the pain is. When an essentially normal physical examination is accompanied by the history of pain and/or cramping of the legs with standing or walking, which are relieved by rest, spinal stenosis should be the number-one suspect in this "crime" of the back. Special tests such as a CAT scan, MRI, or myelogram can determine the presence of spinal stenosis. These tests are described in the section on tests and treatment.

The early treatment for spinal stenosis consists of a back-exercise program and the use of anti-inflammatory medications. Patients are encouraged to engage in activities that do not require extensive walking or running, such as swimming, bicycling, and using a golf cart instead of walking the course. Extra pounds should be shed to help relieve strain on the back. When the pain becomes more debilitating, epidural cortisone injections can provide long-term relief. However, if the pain and limitations persist in spite of all these other measures, surgery can help to relieve the pressure on the nerves. The operation is known as a *decompression laminectomy*, and I will describe it in more detail in the section on treatment.

I have just described three major reasons for low-back pain and related symptoms. However, several other special situations deserve discussion in order to have a comprehensive view of the conditions that can cause back pain. These are problems that are congenital or developmental in nature, result from specific injury, due to arthritis or infection, are related to tumors associated with osteoporosis, and are even a side effect of pregnancy. Two additional causes of back pain will also be discussed: referred pain (pain that feels like it is coming from the back but is not) and psychosomatic pain (where emotional stress and strain play a significant role in the perception of pain).

CONGENITAL

Congenital defects of the spine are an infrequent source of low-back complaints. Congenital anomalies such as spinal bifida, in which the posterior aspect of the vertebral body fails to form, are fortunately very rare. I shall not describe those rare and very serious problems, but rather mention less serious congenital defects that may be associated with back pain, and also describe the developmental problems that can cause pain.

Several times I have mentioned that back-pain sufferers frequently have a family history of such occurrences. Almost invariably, when I question my patients about their family history, I learn that other members of their family have or have had episodes of low-back pain. This is not a "congenital problem" but rather a familial tendency. Many different factors are involved with this familial tendency for back problems.

Congenital defects of the spine that are due to abnormal formation of the bone are in themselves not often sources or causes of low-back pain. As noted earlier, during the formation of the spine, one may have six lumbar vertebrae instead of five, or only four. Occasionally the lowest lumbar vertebra may be totally or partially fused with the sacral segment. Sometimes only half a vertebra is formed, and occasionally vertebrae are even fused together. The L5 and S1 posterior arches may not unite, leaving a spina bifida. About 20 percent of all persons have some congenital variation in the structure of the lower spine. X-rays demonstrate these anomalies, but fortunately most of them are minor deviations and do not cause pain.

Pain in the lower back often can be caused by two related developmental conditions; "developmental" because patients are not born with them, but develop them as they grow. They are *spondylolysis* and *spondylolisthesis*. Although the words may seem formidable and difficult to pronounce, do not be intimidated. Hopefully all you may ever need to know is that they exist.

SPONDYLOLYSIS

If we break down the words into their components, their meaning becomes immediately evident and clear. *Spondylo* refers to the vertebral bone, and *lysis* is to separate or break. Therefore the word means a separation or break in the vertebral bone. The separation or break occurs in the bone bridge between the superior and the inferior facet joints. (See Figure 11.) The bone bridge is called the *pars* (part) *interarticularis* (between two joints). Very logical indeed, as is most medical terminology. All you have to be is a Greek scholar!

Since there is a pars interarticularis on both sides of each vertebra, breaks can occur in one or both bone bridges. When this "break" of the bridge between the facets occurs, an area of instability is created. Motion is possible where previously there was none because the bone was intact. This motion can be painful. The

SPONDYLOLYSIS #11

THE DEFECT OR
SEPARATION IN THE
PARS INTERARTICULARIS

THE DEFECT OR
SEPARATION IN THE
PARS INTERARTICULARIS

break or separation of the bone can occur as the result of chronic or longstanding stress that eventually causes the bridge of bone to give way and separate, or can occur as the result of an acute injury, such as a fracture. Thus, there are two types of spondylolysis. One is acute, resulting from an injury or single event, and the other is a chronic problem that occurs over a long period of time as the bone gives way to constant stress. (If you retain the stretch of an elastic band long enough, it will eventually snap.)

Acute injuries generally occur in young athletes, particularly gymnasts, who are constantly arching or extending their spine with incredible force. This force can actually create a fracture in the pars interarticularis and result in severe back pains and spasms. Special X-rays will reveal the presence of the fracture or spondylolysis. In gymnasts, particularly young girls, the break will occur in the upper portion of the lumbar spine, usually in the L2 or L3 vertebra. Young weight lifters or young high school football players, especially linemen, are also prone to this injury. Fortunately acute spondylolysis can be treated relatively simply with good results by wearing a spinal brace for six to eight weeks.

My nephew developed a spondylolysis while playing high school football. At 142 pounds, he played defensive tackle! At first I ignored his back complaints (the shoemaker's children go without shoes), but one day I watched him limp off the field, twisted and bent over. I knew he had a problem. Special oblique X-rays of the lower spine revealed the spondylolysis. After some grumbling, he agreed to wear a brace for six weeks; fortunately football season was over. His pain subsided. Subsequently he played lacrosse in college without further back problems. One of the things I insisted upon, however, since he did have a "vulnerable back," was that he commit himself to doing back exercises for the rest of his life. I hope he reads this chapter, as a reminder.

The chronic type of spondylolysis is more insidious. The actual break occurs as the result of constant chronic pressure on the pars interarticularis, which slowly causes this bridge of bone to give way and separate. It finally breaks not with a snap, but rather with a sigh (to paraphrase T. S. Eliot). The pains associated with chronic spondylolysis are vague, usually not severe, and generally localized in the back. They may radiate into the buttocks and occasionally even into the thigh, but true sciatic radiation below the knee is not usually present. Muscle spasms and listing of the trunk are concomitant findings. Symptoms tend to be sporadic but eventually culminate in one or more very painful episodes that finally lead to an examination and X-rays.

Chronic spondylolysis breaks typically occur in the L5 vertebra (contradistinction to the acute type, which occurs higher in the lumbar spine). Treatment is essentially the same: bracing until symptoms subside, and a subsequent exercise program. However, the chronic defects are less likely to heal completely. Nevertheless, even if the defect does not heal, the individual may function very well without pain. I advise them to perform the basic exercise program, to modify their athletic activities, and to avoid heavy weight lifting or arching of the back. In a few instances, the pain becomes persistent in spite of conservative treatment and interferes with the person's ability to carry out normal activities. For these individuals, the bony defect can be bridged with bone. In other words, bone fusion or arthrodesis can be performed between the two vertebral bodies, which eliminates motion between the two vertebral segments and thus prevents pain. Obviously surgery is the last resort.

By this time, you may be wondering about that other word I mentioned, *spondylolisthesis*; or maybe you hoped that I would ignore it entirely. As you already know, *spondylo* means "a bone of the spine," specifically a vertebral bone. *Listhesis* means "to slip" or "to displace." When the words are put together— "vertebral bone slip"—you have a visual picture of what happens as one vertebral body slides forward or displaces on another vertebral body. (See Figure 12.) The slip can be just a few degrees, or it can slip entirely off! However, the latter is quite rare.

Why or how does this happen? First, there is a fracture or defect in each pars interarticularis, that bridge of bone that connects the upper and lower facets on both sides of the vertebral body. Once this occurs, the vertebral body is able to slide forward, held back only by the ligaments and intervertebral disks. This condition occurs in about 5 percent of the population, but fortunately most spondylolistheses do not displace too far and can be treated with braces and exercises. The person with this condition has to be carefully followed with periodic X-rays in order to

SPONDYLOLISTHESIS #12

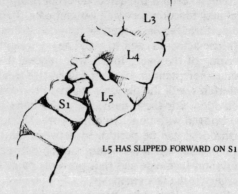

L3

L4

L5

S1

L5 HAS SLIPPED FORWARD ON S1

determine that the slip does not progress. If the slip does progress, the bones must be fused together so that further slippage will be prevented. I shall discuss fusion of bones in greater detail in the section on treatment.

To make the situation even more complicated, there is another condition known as *pseudospondylolisthesis,* which is also a slip or displacement of one vertebral body upon another. In this instance, the pars interarticularis does not fracture or break, but rather elongates, like pulling on taffy. As the elongation occurs, the vertebral body slowly slips forward. Pseudospondylolisthesis is different from the real thing in that there is no actual break and it occurs mainly in older people (sixty or above). Generally pseudospondylolisthesis involves a displacement of the fourth vertebra on the fifth vertebra. The slip is indicative of instability in the localized area, which means that abnormal movements can occur where the slip is present, resulting in back and leg pain. In addition, the canal is narrowed, and symptoms that resemble spinal stenosis can also occur. Has all this been a little too technical and confusing for you? I shall briefly summarize it so you can see the forest and not get lost in the trees.

Spondylolysis is a defect in the bridge of bone that connects the superior and inferior facets of the vertebral body. The defect can be developmental, occurring slowly over a period of time, and usually involves teenagers and young adults. In almost all instances, in the developmental type, it is the L5 vertebral body that is involved. Acute spondylolysis is a similar condition that affects young athletes, particularly gymnasts, weight lifters, and football players, in which a fracture occurs as the result of a traumatic injury in one of the mid- or upper-lumbar vertebra. When a spondylolysis results in one vertebral body sliding forward on another, it becomes a spondylolisthesis. The L5 most commonly slides forward on S1. A pseudospondylolisthesis occurs in older people in whom the pars interarticularis elongates and allows one vertebral body to slide forward upon the other. It is mostly L4 that displaces on L5, but I have even seen L3 slide forward on L4, and L2 on L3.

I hope that you now have a better understanding of these conditions. Remember that they are uncommon causes of low-back and sciatic pain, but must be considered when determining the cause of low-back pain.

OSTEOPOROSIS

A day hardly goes by without an article or some reference in newspapers, magazines, radio, or TV about the condition of *osteoporosis*. This is a major problem for postmenopausal women that rarely affects men. Usually diseases that occur predominantly in one sex more than the other are related to hormonal differences or to genetic patterns. The hormonal difference is especially involved in osteoporosis. After menopause, the levels of estrogen (the female hormone) decrease, and the lack of this substance leads to osteoporosis. Before proceeding further, an explanation of the condition is necessary.

Once again I shall divide the word into its components, which will help clarify the meaning. By now, you know that *osteo* refers to bone and *porosis* is similar to the word *porous*, which means a substance through which water or liquids will flow freely. That is exactly what happens to the bones in women with this problem. Whereas during most of their adult years the bone is densely packed and solid, after menopause, when the estrogen levels fall rapidly, the bones become thinner, less dense, and subsequently not as strong. They are more liable to fracture or to compress from what are considered normal activities. As compression occurs, the height of the vertebral body decreases. (Next time an older person tells you that she is getting shorter, believe her, because when these bones compress, overall body height is decreased. Disk-space narrowing is also a major cause of shortening of the spine.) Most of the collapse occurs in the anterior or front portion of the bone, so that it becomes wedge-shaped—narrower in the front, and higher in the back. This wedge shape occurs in several contiguous bones (most frequently in the dorsal or thoracic spine) and leads to the bent-over or hunched-back attitude seen in older women's spines. Not only does the condition cause disfigurement, but it can also cause significant pain and disability. However, in 65 percent of these patients, the compression fractures happen so gradually that the person has no pain.

For many years, the medical profession had little

treatment to offer for these patients, but intensive research and clinical studies have brought a ray of hope, not only for those who suffer from the disease but also for those who might potentially develop it. In order to understand the treatment of osteoporosis, an explanation of bone content is required.

The vertebral bone is composed of tightly packed thin strands of bone known as *trabeculae*. These trabeculae are made of a protein substance, collagen. Calcium and other minerals are deposited on these collagen fibers, which makes them strong and hard. The trabeculae are held together by a cementlike substance, the matrix. The trabeculae are lined with living bone cells, as are all bones. Specific bone cells constantly resorb old used portions of the trabeculae, and other bone cells add new and healthy bone. After menopause, more bone is resorbed than is replaced, so that instead of being tightly packed it becomes thinner, because each bone contains fewer trabeculae. This "porosity," or lack of bone substance, is readily seen on X-rays of the spine where the decreased density of the bone becomes obvious.

When osteoporosis was first identified as a condition, many doctors felt it was due to chronic and prolonged lack of calcium in the diet. The thinness of the bone on X-rays was interpreted as being due to a lack of calcium. Women were advised to take calcium supplements in large amounts. Unhappily, adding increased amounts of calcium to the diet did not have much helpful effect on these older women. The bones remained thin, weak, and still subject to compression. Additionally the spines of these women would curve even further. The pains would increase in intensity and become constant.

The next advance in treatment of this relentless malady was the use of fluorides. Even little children had learned that brushing their teeth with fluoride would help prevent cavities and keep teeth strong. Well, teeth are like bones, and it was thought that perhaps fluorides could help osteoporosis. Fluorides were given to thousands of women with "thin" bones. It seemed to help slightly. That is, the bones looked thicker and stronger on X-rays, but the trabeculae were still sparse and not thickly packed together. The bone cells were just not producing enough new substance. Finally estrogen was added to the regimen, and that did make a difference. If estrogen was given after menopause, in conjunction with calcium, vitamin D, and fluoride, the quality of the bone was preserved. In women with established osteoporosis, bone density improved, and equally important, the rate of fracture or collapse of the vertebral bodies diminished and pain decreased. Unfortunately, taking estrogen for postmenopausal women is not without risk. Both uterine and breast cancer have been associated with the use of estrogen in postmenopausal women. Before anyone takes estrogen, she should consult both her gynecologist and internist. In a sense, although this combination of treatment is now commonly used, it still remains experimental because its overall effectiveness has not yet been proven.

Prevention is always better than trying to treat the disease, and nowhere is it more important than in women who are premenopausal. There is a definite familial tendency to develop osteoporosis, so if your grandmother or mother has osteoporosis, you are susceptible as well. But don't despair, because you can help yourself. You may not be able to prevent the condition entirely, but you should be able to minimize the problem. Remember that bone is a living and dynamic tissue, which is constantly undergoing resorption and regeneration. Physical stress on bone produced by exercise such as walking, running, bicycling, etc., causes more bone to be produced than is resorbed, thereby retarding the process that produces osteoporosis. Exercise is essential for healthy bones, and helps to prevent osteoporosis in the future.

Calcium supplements can prevent insidious chronic calcium deficiency. A healthy dose of calcium for all women and even men is 1500 mg of calcium a day (as calcium carbonate or preferably calcium citrate). In addition, adding vitamin D, 400 units a day, assures that the calcium is properly absorbed from the intestinal tract.

Throughout the country, osteoporosis centers are being established to help with this problem. Dr. Joseph Lane has established one of the major centers for studies of prevention and treatment of osteoporosis at the Hospital for Special Surgery in New York City. Women are encouraged to have a complete evaluation for osteoporosis whether they are premenopausal or postmenopausal. The evaluation includes blood tests and special X-rays that can measure the density of bones. In addition, an evaluation of the family history and a study of nutritional habits is made. Based upon the results of these studies, it can be determined whether or not osteoporosis is present or whether someone is likely to develop it, and even more important, what might be the best treatment for each individual. Recent reports from major centers reveal that with treatment the incidence of compression fractures of the spine has been reduced by 50 percent and the incidence of hip fractures by 60 percent.

Because of the intensive research that has been done and our new understanding of the treatment of osteoporosis, in the future many millions of women will be saved the collapse of their spines and the agonizing pain that accompanies it. Fifteen years ago, I could not have made such an optimistic statement.

ARTHRITIS

Arthritis is blamed for many ailments and joint pains. The back is no less affected than other parts of the body. How many of you wake up with a "stiff" back in the morning, sort of bent over, with difficulty in straightening up? Well, I am certain that this sign of arthritis is familiar to many of you. What is arthritis, and how does it affect your back?

Let us examine the word for its meanings. *Arthros* means "joint"; *itis* at the end of a word means "infection." Many centuries ago, when the early physicians like Hippocrates and Galen began studying diseases and naming them, they did so without the benefit of X-rays, microscopes, or laboratory tests. They used their five senses—sight, smell, taste, touch, and hearing. For example, they knew about diabetes because the urine of these patients had a distinct odor and a "sweet" taste. We might grimace to think that those old-timers actually tasted urine, but they had to use whatever means were at hand to help them diagnose the problem.

At any rate, these same students of disease looked at a swollen, painful knee and believed it to be infected. They were not able to distinguish between an infection that was caused by a bacteria, virus, or parasite, and an inflammation that was caused by the body's reaction to a noninfectious agent. Hence, over the years the term *arthritis* has come to mean "a chronically painful joint." If you fall and twist your ankle, you have a sprained ankle. If, as years go by, the surface of the joint wears thin as a result of that

66

injury, the joint becomes chronically painful and perhaps even swollen. That is arthritis. Or, more explicitly, that is *osteoarthritis*. Have I complicated it for you by adding the word *osteo* to arthritis? You already know *osteo* means "bones," so now we have created a word that means "bone-joint infection." However, osteoarthritis is due to mechanical wear or tear and is not related to a disease process or to an infection.

Rheumatoid arthritis, on the other hand, is a disease process in which the lining of the joint (the synovium) grows across the surface of the bone ends. The firm, glistening white cartilage, which is on the end of all bones that form a moving joint and allows smooth, almost frictionless motion, is destroyed by this ingrowth of tissue. The cartilage surface becomes eroded and irregular, and bare bone is exposed. When bone rubs against bone, every movement is painful. Thus, rheumatoid and osteoarthritis are very different entities, but both can cause painful joints.

Osteoarthritis is the wearing down of the cartilage on the ends of the bones. This is a natural process of time. Some joints wear down more rapidly because of old injuries that have damaged the joint, or because of a mechanical malalignment. Such is the case with the joints in your back. If there is a malalignment of the joint, pressure on the surfaces is unevenly distributed so that part of the joint gets too much compression, and the other part gets hardly any pressure or wearing at all. The part that gets too much pressure wears out faster, and that is exactly what happens in osteoarthritis. For example, bowed legs are not innocuous. The bowing of the legs puts great stress on the inner or concave side of the knee. Because of the unequal distribution of body weight on the knee, the inner part of the knee joint wears out more rapidly than the outer part. I have simplified the explanation for you.

There are other factors that contribute to the arthritis and to the rapidity with which it develops. Hereditary factors are important. Some families tend to develop osteoarthritis early and more frequently than others, but it is sufficient for you to understand the basic mechanism of osteoarthritis and why it is different from rheumatoid arthritis.

Another term needs defining at this time, and that is *septic arthritis. Septic* indicates an infection, so when we prefix *arthritis* with the word *septic,* we are truly describing an infected joint. The three types of arthritis—rheumatoid, osteo, and septic—can all cause destruction of joints and pains. However, because they are of different etiologies, or causes, their treatment will be different as well. Rheumatoid arthritis can be treated with certain medications, including cortisone preparations and anti-inflammatory medications. Septic arthritis can be treated with antibiotics. Osteoarthritis can sometimes be treated with anti-inflammatory medications to reduce pain, but basically the thrust of treatment is to preserve muscle strength around the joint and to try to correct malalignment.

If you get out of bed in the morning with a stiff back and have difficulty straightening up, but after a while, perhaps after a hot shower, you find that you are straighter and moving about with less difficulty, you may indeed have a touch of osteoarthritis of your spine. Osteoarthritis of the spine is not curable, but, as noted, the pain that is often associated with it can be relieved with anti-inflammatory medications. Mobility and strength can be maintained with exercises.

The symptoms of rheumatoid arthritis can also be relieved with various medications. There are several types of rheumatoid arthritis that involve the spine. There is a special variant of the disease in young men known as *ankylosing spondylitis,* in which the vertebral bodies become bound together by bony overgrowth. The spine becomes stiff and rigid. It is often painful, but medications can help to relieve the pain. Eventually, when the spine is totally rigid, the pain eases. Special blood tests can help determine the presence of this disease.

I have taken you through this rather lengthy explanation of arthritis in order to tell you about arthritis of the spine. All three types of arthritis can occur in your back—osteo, rheumatoid, or septic arthritis. However, the latter two are very rare, whereas osteoarthritis is much more common, especially among older individuals who have had more "wear and tear" on their spines, though not all older people develop osteoarthritis.

PREGNANCY AND BACK PAIN

Without pregnancy and birth, the human race would cease to exist. Why, then, was the process not made easier and at least free from back pain? I cannot answer that question, but I certainly can testify that back pain is a frequent annoyance and sometimes an agony of pregnancy. The majority of women are not troubled by their backs during pregnancy, but a number of them are, and over the years I have treated hundreds of pregnant women complaining of their aching backs.

Often the problem exists before they even become pregnant—that is, their backs were not in great shape (from an orthopedic point of view, at any rate) before that miraculous moment when their pregnancy began.

The pregnant state causes significant changes in a woman's body. The initial hormone changes that can cause drowsiness and fatigue as well as the familiar "morning sickness" diminish the endurance of the muscles that support the spine. As the pregnancy advances, the fetus enlarges, and the abdomen becomes disproportionately large, and in order to compensate, women lean backward, thereby increasing their lumbar lordosis and producing greater stresses upon their lower backs. (See Figure 13.) Toward the end of the pregnancy, hormones are secreted that soften the ligaments that hold the pelvic bones together, thus preparing the birth canal for the expansion necessary in order for the baby to be born. These same hormones similarly affect the ligaments of the spine, which are already under abnormal stress due to the increased lordosis. If these ligaments are stretched even further, it produces additional strain on the muscles and joints of the lower back. These increased stresses cause pain, and on occasion can injure a disk in the lower back.

Many women complain of radiating pain in their legs in the last few weeks of pregnancy. This sciatic type of pain may be due to the pressure of the baby actually lying on the nerve, or it may be due to a bulging or rupture of a disk secondary to the excessive strain on the lower back. Unfortunately, if the pain is severe, the only remedy is bed rest. After the baby is born, the pain subsides, except in those rare individuals in whom the disk had actually herniated or ruptured. Then the pain will persist for many weeks or even months. Sometimes surgery is necessary to excise the slipped disk. With this sobering thought, allow me to relieve the sense of doom by reiterating the common message throughout this book.

Exercises to keep your back healthy before, during, and after pregnancy can avoid these problems. Obstetricians recognize the need to maintain good muscle tone in the body for a healthier pregnancy and easier delivery. Attending prenatal exercise classes is a must, not only for the expectant mother, but also for the

PREGNANT WOMAN #13

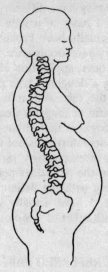

expectant father. Not that proud Daddy can make his wife's pregnancy easier by strengthening his own back, but at least he can be supportive and encouraging, which provides an emotional lift for his wife.

Many pregnant patients have told me that they are afraid to do exercises for fear of harming the baby, especially in the last trimester of pregnancy. Postural recumbent exercises with slight modifications are safe for the baby and very helpful for the mother's back. Always consult your obstetrician before starting the exercises, and confer with him regularly about the exercises as your pregnancy continues.

Once the baby is born, your problems are over, right? Well, maybe not. During delivery of a baby, a great deal of force is exerted upon the coccyx, the tailbone. Sometimes this bone becomes very inflamed and tender. You may have difficulty sitting or getting up from a chair. I have even seen patients in whom the coccyx has actually been broken during delivery, but that is a very rare occurrence. Usually the pain will resolve with time, application of ice, avoidance of pressure by using a doughnut-type pillow to sit upon, and soaking in the tub. Anti-inflammatory medications such as aspirin or ibuprofen can also be helpful. A comforting thought is that although the coccyx can cause pain and discomfort, it is not usually a disabling problem. Except in exceedingly rare cases, it always gets better. When the pain does persist and becomes chronic, interfering with the patient's ability to carry on a normal life, I have actually excised this small piece of bone, with relief of symptoms.

REFERRED PAIN

Question: When is a back pain not a back pain? Answer: When it comes from somewhere else. I have already cited examples of referred pain arising from other parts of the body—heart, kidney, and gallbladder —so they need not be repeated here. What concerns us now is how we can differentiate pains felt in the back, but that do not originate in the spine.

How do we explain this phenomenon of referred pain? It is complex and not entirely understood, but the basic premise is that two or more nerves may share a common pathway to carry sensation to our brain. These messages are interpreted "en masse" to the brain, and some distinctions become blurred. In addition, nerves from different parts of the body may end up at the same brain location, which causes further confusion. Thus, a person having a heart attack and experiencing chest pain may also be aware of pain in the left arm. The two have a common pathway, and stimulation of one stimulates the other.

Referred pain to the back works in the same fashion. Damage of adjacent organs such as the kidneys, uterus, and prostate can refer pain to the back.

Several times a year, a patient will be referred to my office because of back pain, and upon examination I find that the back is normal but the pain is arising from another source. For instance, a young man of forty had pain in his back and hip that kept him awake at night. The only relief he had was when he took a hot bath. He walked into my office with an erect posture, and had no pain when I asked him to twist and bend his spine. When I gently tapped his back, just below the ribs, he cried out in pain. His spine was fine, but he had a kidney infection that caused the pain in his back. Appropriate antibiotics (prescribed by his internist) cured his back pain, and fortunately his kidney infection as well.

Another example of referred pain is the older lady who presented with right-leg sciatic pain. The pain had been present for several weeks, but was getting so bad that she could barely walk a block. She also complained of numbness and frequent pins and needles in her feet. She brought X-rays to my office that revealed moderate arthritic changes in her lumbar spine. On examination, she did have mild stiffness in her lower back. Her right foot felt colder than her left, but that is occasionally seen with sciatica. The most important finding was that the pulses in her right foot were barely felt, and the pulses in her left foot were normal. That difference suggested a circulatory problem, and when the proper tests were done, she was discovered to have a partial blockage of the blood flow to her right leg. Removal of the blockage relieved her symptoms.

These two case histories emphasize the need for thorough evaluation of all back and leg pain. We should not be quick to make a diagnosis of a back problem until we have all the facts.

The most important aspect of referred pain is to know that it exists. The doctor who takes care of your back will thoroughly evaluate your symptoms, and with his examination should be able to determine whether it is your back or something else causing your pain. The next time you have back pain, it might be wise for you to consider the possibility of the pain being referred from elsewhere and pay attention to other parts of your body.

EMOTIONAL STRESS ON THE BACK

I debated whether this section should come first or last in this chapter. Some doctors are convinced that 80 percent of all back pain is psychosomatic or stress-related. In the mid-eighties, I discussed this problem with a well-known New York doctor on television. This doctor insisted that 80 percent of all back problems were related to emotional stress, and he had an elaborate theory to explain why muscles go into spasm as a result of this type of stress. The cure for back problems, he believes, is in the recognition that they are caused by emotional stress. That is, when you know your back pain is stress-related, you can help yourself reduce the stress and thus relieve the pain. My viewpoint was that 80 percent of the patients had some mechanical or organic problem with their back, and that only 20 percent of the problems were psychologically induced.

How could such disparate views exist? In this instance, both of us were recognized as experts in our field and respected by our peers and the community. How could we sit there and make exactly opposite statements? We both couldn't be right. Or could we? Well, let us examine the patient population that we treat. Both of us work in New York City, a highly urban, stressful environment. No differences there. However, Dr. S. is known for his theories about emotional stress and back pain, and I am known for my emphasis on the treatment of organic or mechanical back pains by exercise programs. New patients are referred to my office by other doctors and other patients. The same is true for Dr. S. This pattern of patient referral is inherently selective, so that 80 percent of the patients I examine have mechanical problems with their backs, and 80 percent of the patients Dr. S. examines have psychological stress problems with their backs. So we may both be right in recording what we experience in our practices.

Not for one moment do I minimize the importance of stress on the production of pain. But I do believe that there is a vast difference between physical stress affecting weak back structures and emotional stress in which pain is the result of psychological problems.

The word *stress* has many implications, and I shall define it as it relates to back problems. There is physical stress and there is emotional stress. Physical stress is the tension or pressure that is put upon finite objects. The hurricane stressed the trees in its path, and many trees bent and broke. The weight lifter stressed every muscle in his body as he set about establishing a new record. That type of stress is easy to comprehend. We have all strained and stressed our bodies physically. Lifting too much or twisting while holding a heavy weight are stresses that can cause back pain.

Emotional stress is less easy to define, yet we are all aware of it. In fact, statements like "he is really stressed out" have become part of our everyday vocabulary. Emotional stresses are common to all people. No one can avoid them, and in today's highly industrialized urban-oriented world, these stresses are greater than ever, while people have a decreased ability to relieve their individual tensions.

Stress is a natural phenomenon in all animals and is related to the way we react to danger in our environment. When a deer hears a strange noise or catches an unusual scent in the air, its ears quiver, its eyes get bigger, and a rush of adrenaline through its body prepares it for flight. When the phone rings late at night, I awake with a start, my heart begins to pound, and I anticipate bad news. The rise in my pulse rate prepares my body for the stress of that bad news.

Just think for a moment of all the trying things that happened to you today. How do you deal with stress? Activity usually helps. A good cry can relieve stress, but we are not always able to cry in front of other people. Shouting and venting your anger helps. Blanking out the environment with television or a book distracts your mind and emotions. Some people sleep long hours to blot out problems and stresses. But more and more people are engaging in aerobic-type exercise programs that not only improve their muscle tone and their cardiopulmonary function, but also burn off that excess adrenaline that circulates in the body as a result of all the stresses they have encountered during the day. Exercise has become our most important method of not only keeping our bodies, hearts, and lungs strong, but also of relieving inner tensions.

After that rather long discussion, how does stress relate to your back? If you have back problems of any sort and you have neglected them, the muscles in your back are generally weak. Thus, when you are under tension and stress and your muscles are "tight," especially your back muscles, they are more likely to fatigue quickly and go into spasm. That is one way in which stress can directly produce low-back pain. Obviously this stress occurs over a period of time, perhaps days, weeks, or even months before the spasm occurs and the pain hits you.

One of my patients recently made a statement that is simple yet profound. He told me that he finally realized the significance of the term *"a pain in the ass."* This patient, a successful middle-aged businessman, had had intermittent low-back pain with sciatica many years ago. Often the pain would linger in his buttock region and become very annoying, especially while he was sitting. This gentleman was a very disciplined individual who did exercises faithfully every day. He boasted about being free of pain for many years, able to play golf, tennis, and fish without a thought or worry. Then, two weeks before he came to my office, he began having difficulty with sitting and experienced annoying pain in his lower back with persistant radiation into his buttocks. He tried to work it out with exercises. The pains became worse. He rested in bed, he took medications, and the pains persisted.

Finally he came for an examination. I had known him for over ten years, and had actually operated upon his back to remove a herniated disk. His recovery from that surgery was splendid, and he was a paragon of diligence in doing his back exercises. We were both happy and pleased with his progress. What happened? Why this sudden onset of pain after being pain-free for so long and being so diligent with his exercises? Was it a new disk herniation? Something out of alignment in his back? After examination and X-rays, I was able to conclude that there was no new disk herniation and nothing out of whack in his back.

But he did have muscle spasm, and he did have typical sciatica with a very real "pain in the ass." So we sat down and talked.

I learned that he had been under a great deal of stress the past few months. He was exercising, but not really as often or as thoroughly as he once did. He was traveling a great deal, especially on planes, and sitting for long hours flying from one coast to the other on overnight trips. He was not sleeping as well or as long. To top it all off, his daughter was having serious marital problems with her husband. He said he was fine, but was he?

The situation is all too familiar. He had successfully recovered from back surgery for a herniated disk. He was doing his back exercises faithfully and also enjoying other general exercises. He knew the basic mechanics of back care and avoided unnecessary strains on his back, but with time he got careless, less concerned, and gradually paid less attention to his back. And suddenly, after a period of a few months, he was placed under great stress, traveling a great deal and getting too little sleep. Inevitably the old weak area of the back finally gave out, and the long-forgotten pain recurred. There are two morals to this story. First, you never really cure a back problem, you only control it, and that control requires a lifelong effort. Second, even if you do the proper exercises for your back, excessive stress and fatigue can be your undoing. The back-exercise program in this book can keep your muscles strong and protect your back, but emotional stress and fatigue over an extended time can still cause problems. Just as your back needs strong muscles to be healthy, so do your body and mind need an outlet for your emotional stress.

For this individual, I pointed out the need for recreational activities that would not only provide an outlet to release his inner tensions, but also remove him physically from his stress-producing environments, the home and office. Naturally I reinforced the need for him to continue his daily back exercises. I also recommended that he should not be reluctant to seek professional help for assistance in relieving his inner tensions.

Psychosomatic pain is different from pain caused by stress. This pain is perceived as real by the patient and is in the general region of the lower back or legs. However, these patients tend to exaggerate their symptoms. They describe excruciating pain while smiling. They tell me that they cannot sit for more than ten minutes, yet seem to be comfortable sitting and describing in great detail all the nuances of their pain. At times they describe symptoms that I know are anatomically impossible to produce. Are they lying? Malingering? Is there a liability or compensation lawsuit involved? Is the patient deliberately trying to mislead me, to make me believe the disability is worse than it is in order to make a pile of money in a settlement? These are hard questions to answer. Fortunately, in almost thirty years of practice, I have had very few people who I felt were deliberately lying about their symptoms for litigation purposes.

However, I have seen dozens of people whose symptoms are exaggerated due to emotional stress. Having a "bad back" is an accepted way to avoid dealing with unpleasant situations. For example, there is the nurse who always gets back pains when she has the night shift because she hates to work nights. It is not a deliberate event, but rather because she becomes so stressed and depressed by working nights that her "back" acts up. Or there is the truck driver whose home life is tension-packed with an alcoholic wife and unruly children, who gets back spasms in South Carolina and can't get home to New Jersey for several days. The young man with great insecurities has difficulty making decisions, and when he is faced with the need to make a significant decision, he winds up in the hospital in traction with a bad back—the decision deferred and perhaps made by someone else. And so it goes.

People who have real emotional problems and crises often develop physical outlets for their inner anguish and pain. Some people develop migraine headaches, others asthma, some ulcers, and some develop back pain. These people have back pain that cannot be relieved until their emotional needs are helped, and we know that that is not always possible. I find it easier to treat someone with an organic/mechanical back problem than someone with a functional or emotional back problem. For the former, I can prescribe medication or exercises with very good expectations of affording them relief. For the latter, I try to support them emotionally, give them a sense of my caring and concern, but I cannot change the social, economic, and psychological factors in their lives that are the true initiating causes of their pain. After all that, I repeat what I said earlier: Eighty percent of all the back patients I see have an organic or mechanical reason for their symptoms, often aggravated by stress. The other 20 percent have an emotional etiology of their pain. Both groups need help.

LESS COMMON CAUSES OF BACK PAIN: FRACTURES, INFECTIONS, TUMORS

To be complete but not painstakingly so, I need to include a brief discussion about some unusual causes of back pain. These are generally more serious problems, and I mention them only to differentiate these conditions from the more usual everyday stress of mechanical back pains. I shall discuss fractures (not as ominous as they sound), infections, and tumors of the spine.

Fractures

A bone has not been made that cannot be broken or fractured, and this is also true of the vertebrae. The two words, *broken* or *fractured,* mean the same thing and are interchangeable. Naturally, when you hear that someone has a fractured spine, it is a cause of great concern. The danger of paralysis from a broken spine is all too evident, especially after you have learned how closely the spinal cord is related to its protective bony cover. Severe fractures with displacement can cause sufficient injury to the spinal cord to result in paralysis. If the injury is in the neck, it can result in *quadriplegia,* where the paralysis involves all four limbs. If it occurs in the dorsal or lumbar spine, *paraplegia* occurs, paralyzing the person from the waist down. Unfortunately a severed or crushed spinal cord cannot be repaired and does not regenerate; the paralysis is permanent. Although some spinal injuries to the cord may only be a contusion or compression injury, they can have disastrous outcomes if prompt treatment is not undertaken. There is no need to describe these dramatic problems to you in detail. The diagnosis is evident after a serious injury, and treatment is always carried out in the hospital.

There are fractures of the spinal bones that occur as the result of injury and cause pain, but may not be readily recognized and diagnosed. A typical fracture of the spine is a compression fracture of the vertebral body. Mrs. S. is hanging a picture on her wall and is standing on a rickety chair that topples over. She falls backward and "fortunately" lands on her bottom. She experiences pain but is relieved that she did not land on her head. Her lower back is sore, and gradually she develops stiffness in her lower back, with difficulty getting in and out of a chair. That night she takes aspirin for the pain, but whenever she attempts to turn over in bed, she still has sharp spasms of pain. By the next morning, she can barely get out of bed. The pain in her lower back is agonizing. She wisely calls her physician for an examination. X-rays are taken of her lower back, and on careful inspection, a compression fracture of the L1 vertebra is observed.

This is a common event. Falling from a height, landing on the buttocks or even on the feet, exerts a tremendous compression force upon the spine. This force asserts its maximum power at the junction of the dorsal spine, which is relatively immobile, and the lumbar spine, which is relatively flexible. With the impact of the fall, slight flexion of the trunk usually occurs, and the anterior surfaces of T12 and L1 vertebra are slammed together, resulting in a compression of either T12 or L1 or both. Wait, you may ask, if the fracture is at T12 or L1, why does Mrs. S. complain of pain in the lower back in the L5 and S1 region? The answer to that is "referred pain." Indeed, the pain in the upper region is referred to the lower-back region. Careful palpation can reveal the real source of pain. Pressure applied to the T12 or L1 region will be painful. X-rays should always include the dorsal spine as well as the lumbar spine after any type of back injury.

Most of these fractures are not serious. They heal well in about six to eight weeks. Treatment is usually bed rest until the acute pain subsides, and then the use of a lightweight spinal brace. With exercises, the patient can return to normal daily activities but should avoid any strenuous exercises or lifting for about three to four months. Older people, especially postmenopausal women, are prone to compression fractures of the spine. Because of osteoporosis, these fractures can result from relatively minor trauma.

You may wonder how Mrs. S. managed to get around at all after her fall and while sustaining a "broken spine." Well, as I indicated, the compression fracture is not a typical broken bone. Although the bone is fractured, the posterior elements of the vertebral bone remain intact, and as long as these structures are intact, the spinal cord is protected. If the fracture extends through the vertebral body into the spinal canal, then the spinal cord is in danger of being injured. But still, you may persist, how could she even manage to stand up after that fracture?

I am often amazed at the ability of people to withstand pain. Several years ago, I had the great privilege and pleasure of treating a very distinguished U.S. senator. He had been on a wilderness trip with a group of friends. One of the obstacles this group had to overcome was a jump from a thirty-foot cliff into a deep river. For someone who had been in the parachute troops in the Second World War, this was a simple exercise. However, even an old pro can make a mistake. He hit the water awkwardly, misjudging the time of impact, and his trunk flexed forward. He experienced a sharp stabbing pain in his back that took his breath away. He forced himself to relax, and somehow swam to the opposite shore. When he rested for a while, he was able to get up, put on his backpack, and trek the remainder of the day, albeit in considerable pain. His discomfort was obvious to his companions, although he tried to conceal how bad it was. Since they were flying back through New York City, one of his friends called and asked if I could see him as soon as they arrived.

He walked into my office with a warm, friendly smile, and apologized for intruding upon my time. I could see he had difficulty moving about and changing positions. His neurological examination was entirely normal. He had marked tenderness in the upper-lumbar region, and sure enough, the X-rays confirmed that he had a compression fracture of L1. Imagine swimming out of a river, walking over rough terrain with a backpack, and flying in a plane for five hours with a fracture of the spine! What courage, what a fine example of the inner strength that exists in all of us when we need it. I advised a back brace for eight weeks, after which he began the exercise program. I am pleased to report that the senator has had a complete recovery and is as active and as vigorous as ever, without back pain.

Infections

In the modern antibiotic era, infections of the spine are quite uncommon. When tuberculosis was rampant, spinal involvement was frequent and often devastating. That infection would literally destroy the vertebral bones, cause large collections of pus, and often result in irreversible destruction of the spinal cord. The dorsal spine was most often involved with this dreaded disease, but the cervical and lumbar spine were not spared. Today, tuberculosis and other bacterial infections of the spine are quite rare. However, they do occur, and doctors must be alert to that possibility.

The sequence and type of symptoms provide valuable clues that the pain may be a result of an infection of the vertebral bones. The onset of pain is very gradual, and then suddenly becomes very intense. Severe intermittent muscle spasms may be present. The patient may have a fever or sweat profusely at night. The spine is very tender to touch or pressure.

Blood tests reveal an increase in white blood cells, and the ESR is elevated. X-rays may be negative in the early stages of the infection, but after three to four weeks, infection in the bone can be seen. A bone scan would be positive early in the course of the disease. (See the chapter on tests for explanation of these terms.)

Treatment requires hospitalization and identification of the organism causing the infection. Once the diagnosis is made, appropriate intravenous antibiotic treatment is given. Subsequently a spinal brace is worn until complete healing of the involved bones is achieved. Happily almost all infections of the spine can be successfully treated this way. Occasionally surgery may be necessary to help remove infected material. The earlier a diagnosis is made and the sooner antibiotics are started, the better will be the outcome. Fortunately the sophisticated testing that exists today facilitates the early diagnosis of spinal bone infections.

Tumors

Cancer is on everyone's mind, and nearly all of us have contact with someone who has cancer and may be dying of the disease. We are concerned about pain and worry that it may be the presenting sign of cancer. Certainly many of my back patients have expressed that fear to me or voiced their relief after I examined them and diagnosed "something simple," like a herniated disk. It is a natural anxiety, and tumors of the spine can cause back pain. You are probably aware that not all tumors are cancerous, and that some tumors are designated "benign" because they do not invade local tissues or spread to other parts of the body. Malignant tumors, on the other hand, do invade local tissues and can spread to elsewhere in the body. Benign tumors of the spine can cause pain, but are rare. If they are readily accessible, they can be surgically removed; otherwise they are left alone as long as the pressure of their presence does not cause compression of the spinal cord or result in fracture of the bone.

Malignant tumors or cancers are more ominous. They can either arise locally, primarily from the vertebral body itself, or metastasize (spread) to the spine from another site. The cancers that most commonly spread to the spine usually come from the lung, prostate, thyroid, breast, or kidney.

Treatment of spinal cancers depends upon the type of tumor and whether or not it originates in the vertebral bones or comes from another site. Since treatment of spinal tumors and cancers is not pertinent to this book, we will not deal with them further. As you are aware, radiation, chemotherapy, and even surgery all play a role in their treatment.

The symptoms of cancer of the spine are different from those of the usual backache. The pain is constant, nagging, gradually becoming worse. Whereas most back patients can ease their pain by lying down, patients with cancer of the spine have pain even while in bed. Whenever patients tell me they cannot sleep because of back pain, I become suspicious and order special tests for in-depth evaluation of these symptoms.

My final word on cancers of the spine is to remind you that they are not common, in fact they are very rare. Don't allow yourself to become so anxious about the possibility of cancer that your back pain grows worse. The likelihood that you have cancer of the spine is very small indeed.

DIAGNOSING YOUR BACK PAIN

After reading through these several early chapters, you might feel qualified to make specific diagnoses yourself. Do not do that. Remember, a little knowledge can be a dangerous thing. My purpose in writing this book is not to make you an instant qualified doctor, but rather to make you aware of the various problems that an unhealthy back can cause and to show you how to avoid these problems by building a healthy back.

I hope you have learned so far how to distinguish the different types of pain—localized to the lower back, radiating into the leg, and the cramping sensations of the legs associated with spinal stenosis. I also hope that you realize the need for medical attention when the pain is really bad or persists beyond a few days.

The first time you have back pain, you do not have to run to a specialist such as an orthopedic surgeon, neurologist, or neurosurgeon. I strongly recommend that you see your family physician first. He or she is qualified to give you an overall examination and evaluation. If the doctor feels the need for further consultation, he will refer you to the appropriate specialist. Another advantage of seeing your family doctor or internist first is that he or she can evaluate your general condition and make certain that your pain is not referred.

4. Tests and Treatment

The physical examination has been completed, and I have told you briefly about the structure of the back and the pains and tribulations that can occur as the result of having a back problem. It is now time to look at the positive side of things and talk about the tests and treatments available to ease your pains and make your life enjoyable once more.

TESTS

If you have already had X-rays and blood tests, then further tests may not be necessary, but as this is your first visit for your back problem, I may take certain blood tests and standard X-rays of your spine. I emphasize *may*, because if I feel that you have primarily a muscular problem, X-rays may not be necessary.

There is nothing wrong in recommending to a patient that X-rays be deferred. If the pain subsides promptly, then you have saved the patient time, money, and radiation exposure. If the pain persists, then X-rays can be taken safely one or even two weeks later. The purpose of these routine X-rays of the spine is to evaluate the spinal bones.

From standard X-rays, I can determine if the spine is straight, I can see evidence of arthritis, and I can diagnose fractures. But I cannot see a slipped disk or inflamed nerve root. These soft tissues, as opposed to the hard tissues like bone, are not visible on routine X-rays. I may infer that a disk is damaged by the presence of narrowing of the space between the two intervertebral bodies. When the disk is damaged or degenerated, it collapses, and then the space between the bone is visibly narrowed on X-ray. However, the narrowing does not necessarily mean a disk herniation. It could be just a degeneration within the disk itself. Spondylolysis and spondylolisthesis can also be diagnosed with X-rays, although special side and oblique views are often necessary to see the defect clearly.

Of course, any congenital abnormalities of the bone can also be determined on X-ray, four or six instead of five lumbar vertebrae, for example. A disk space may be absent entirely, with the bones being fused together; or spina bifida, a defect in the posterior elements in the spinous process, may also be observed. These conditions themselves may not be the cause of back problems, but it is important to know that they are present, and they have to be considered as part of the overall evaluation of the patient. More often than not, the back X-rays are "normal" or "negative," but that does not rule out the possibility of a herniated disk or other soft-tissue problems.

Specific tests are ordered for specific problems, not as part of a routine evaluation. Five special X-ray tests are frequently employed to help in the diagnosis of back problems. They are the CT or CAT scan, the MRI (magnetic resonance imaging), myelograms, diskograms, and bone scans.

NO MORE ACHING BACK

CT (Computerized Axial Tomography)

The CT or CAT scan has been a great help in evaluating what goes on in our bodies. It can present a three-dimensional image of your internal structures to show views that were previously not possible using the standard X-ray. With a routine X-ray, we can see only the side and front of the vertebral columns, but with the CT scan we can see a cross section of the area. We can even visualize the spinal cord and nerve roots. With the CT scan, a herniated disk becomes visible. Although the CT scan is enormously helpful, there are limits to what it can depict. It is an X-ray technique, and the patient does receive small amounts of radiation. Bony details are well demonstrated on the CT scans. Spinal stenosis (narrowing of the central canal, and narrowing of the nerve-root exits) can be nicely visualized on these images.

MRI (Magnetic Resonance Imaging)

This new, miraculous method of looking into our bodies is done without the aid of radiation. Essentially you lie within an enormous magnet, which attracts electrical charges from your body—charges normally present in everyone. An ultra-fine computer collects all these impulses and then reconstructs images of the area of the body that is being investigated. Because this test does not rely upon radiation beams, even soft tissues can be visualized on the film, which looks just like an X-ray film. We can see cross-sectional views of the spinal-cord area, and also see side views of the spine. If a herniated disk is compressing the dura or spinal cord, this can also be visualized on the MRI. While the CT scan is usually better for bony definition, the MRI shows the soft tissues more clearly.

A major drawback of the MRI is that you have to

lie inside a big tube for forty-five to sixty minutes. People with claustrophobia are unable to tolerate that. In addition, the MRI is a very expensive test.

Myelogram

Probably the most feared and maligned procedure in the diagnosis of back problems is the myelogram. This is a test in which a needle is inserted into the lower back and into the dura or covering of the spinal cord. Several drops of spinal fluid are extracted and sent for routine analysis. Then a colorless liquid (a dye) is injected into the space around the nerve roots and spinal cord. On an X-ray image, dense materials appear "lighter" and the less-dense structures appear "darker." For example, air, which is the least dense of all substances, appears completely black on X-rays. Muscles may appear grayish, whereas bone is whitish. The myelogram is done with X-ray controls on a special X-ray table. In most hospitals, it is done by a radiologist. However, in some areas neurologists and even orthopedic surgeons do their own myelograms. In our hospital, the procedure is done by our radiologists.

Once the dye has been injected, the patient is moved from side to side, and X-rays are taken. Then the table is tilted up and down to encourage a flow of the dye within the spinal canal, and further X-rays are taken. The column of dye can be moved up to the neck or cervical region if interpretation of this area is necessary.

Many years ago an oil-based dye was used that had to be removed at the end of the procedure. This was often painful and a major reason that myelograms were dreaded. Today, the dye is a water-soluble substance that can be resorbed through the membranes of the spinal cord and finally excreted in the urine. This has simplified the procedure, made it more comfortable for the patient, and at the same time has given better definition and a clearer view of the inside of the spinal canal.

With the advent of the CT and MRI, myelograms are not as essential as they once were. However, when the diagnosis remains obscure, or the exact degree of disk herniation cannot be determined, the myelogram is still the most accurate test. This is especially true when a CT scan is done with the dye still in the spinal column. Today, I routinely follow a myelogram with a CT scan.

The ill effects of the water-soluble myelogram are few. Headaches and nausea occur only occasionally afterward. Drinking copious amounts of fluid prior to the myelogram helps to prevent that complication. I generally recommend that patients be admitted to the hospital the night before the myelogram in order to have IV fluids so that they are well hydrated (filled with water) before the procedure. The excess water in the system dilutes the dye material as it enters the bloodstream and hastens its departure from the body in the urine. By the way, after the myelogram is completed, you will be asked to sit up in bed for eight hours in order to keep the dye in the lower part of your back and prevent it from flowing up to your head, where it can cause headaches, nausea, and vomiting.

Almost always, when I recommend that patients have a myelogram, there is an instant reaction of fear and anxiety. Someone always knows someone else who had a bad reaction to that test. I try to reassure and calm patients' fears because while they almost invariably are anxious about the impending procedure, after it is over they invariably say it was easy and did not hurt. They then wonder why so many people said it would be awful.

I hope I have reassured you if you ever need to have a myelogram, but remember, a myelogram is not done unless you are not responding to treatment or the results of a CT or MRI are not conclusive.

Diskogram

Once in a while even sophisticated tests such as CT scan, MRI, or myelogram may be negative or inconclusive, and yet there is still a strong suspicion on a doctor's part that the problems may be coming from a herniated disk. In these cases, a diskogram may be very helpful.

A diskogram is an X-ray procedure in which a needle is actually inserted into the intervertebral disk. This is performed with X-ray control, usually by the radiologist, but again often done by neurologists or orthopedic surgeons. When the X-ray confirms that the tip of the needle has been inserted within the disk, a few drops of "dye" are injected into the area. In a normal disk, the dye stays within the central portion of the disk, the nucleus-pulposus area. If the disk has ruptured through the annulus fibrosis, the material will leak out from the disk space. If the disk is bulging, it will just leak into the area where it is bulging. Diskograms can be done on outpatients. That is, most of the time patients do not have to be admitted to the hospital to have the procedure done.

Bone Scans

The purpose of a bone scan is to measure the activity of the cells in the bones of the spine. It also helps to determine if something seen on the X-ray is of recent origin or old. First, I'll explain what a bone scan is, and then I'll tell you what we learn from it.

A bone scan requires an injection of a liquid into your vein, usually the vein in front of your elbow. This does not hurt more than the usual needle for a blood test. The material injected is "radioactive." That is, it emits an electric-like impulse. Fortunately the radioactivity soon diminishes, and there is little or no danger from it. In fact, the Food and Drug Administration has approved its use for children. This material is carried around the body by the bloodstream, and as it passes through bones, it is absorbed into the bone cells. Normal bone collects only a small portion of the circulating *ions,* as they are called. Dead bone doesn't collect any of the ions, and bone that is hyperactive due to an infection, fracture, or tumor picks up large amounts of the ions.

Two hours after the injection, the patient is asked to lie on the table under a Geiger counter, a machine that records radioactivity. This Geiger counter passes over the body and records the amount of radioactivity in each area. The information is then fed into a computer that analyzes it and presents an outline of the human body with tiny dots. In areas where blood circulation is poor or the bone is dead, these dots are absent, and these areas appear "white." Where the bone cells are hyperactive and circulation increased, these dots are densely packed, appearing as solid dark areas. These dark areas are what are known as "hot spots" because they indicate a high concentration of the radioactive ions. This type of activity is not recorded by a CT scan, MRI, or myelogram, so that the bone scan provides different information from those other tests. For instance, if a compression fracture of a vertebral body is seen on X-rays, a bone scan can tell us whether it is a recent or old event. If it is an old event and the bone is already healed, the concentration of spots will appear normal. If it is recent and still healing, the bone scan would indicate a "hot spot." A bone scan may detect the presence of a fracture in the pars interarticularis (spondylolysis) which may not be visible on the routine X-rays. Bone scans also show arthritis of the spine. And yes, bone scans can also reveal the presence of a tumor in the spine. If your doctor orders a bone scan of your spine, do not become overly fearful. As you can see, there are many conditions other than cancer for which he may be looking.

Blood Tests

Since most back pain and sciatica are the result of mechanical problems, such as instability or a herniated disk, blood tests are not usually necessary for diagnostic purposes. However, if an infection or arthritis is being considered, then blood tests are very important. Probably 90 percent of back problems fall into the group of patients that do not require blood tests. The physician is always aware of rare causes of back pain, and if the history or physical examination raises any doubts or suspicions, then in addition to the X-rays (which I've already discussed), appropriate blood tests should be ordered. Usually I order three different tests: a routine blood count, a blood-chemistry profile, and an erythrocyte-sedimentation rate (ESR).

A routine blood count measures the number of red and white cells in your bloodstream. The red cells carry oxygen, and the white cells fight infections. If the number of red cells is decreased, your body is receiving less oxygen, and you are anemic. If the number of white cells is increased, you probably have an infection or inflammation or both of these somewhere in your body.

The blood-chemistry profile is another screening test for evaluation of liver and kidney function, muscle enzymes, calcium and phosphorous levels, and also blood-urea nitrogen and uric acid. Uric-acid-level tests are done to determine the presence or absence of gout. If the uric acid is high, then gout is probably present, and gout can cause pain not only in the great toe but also in the back. Calcium-blood levels are an important indicator of body metabolism. If the calcium levels are either too low or too high, it is usually related to a metabolic disorder.

The ESR or erythrocyte-sedimentation rate is a test that also indicates the presence of an inflammation or infection in the body. The fire alarm signals smoke, but does not indicate whether the smoke comes from a cigarette or a blazing fire in the living room. Similarly the ESR indicates that there is something wrong, but does not provide a specific diagnosis.

Other special blood tests are helpful in diagnosing arthritis. As I mentioned earlier, there are several different types of arthritis. Osteoarthritis cannot be determined by blood tests. However, there are several tests that are concerned with septic and rheumatoid arthritis or its variants. When a doctor orders these tests for you, he will probably say that he is ordering blood tests for arthritis, but he may not describe the specific tests. Actually those are details you really don't have to know. Just be aware that the tests are being ordered for the possibility of arthritis.

Special Neurological Tests:
EMG and Nerve-Conduction Studies

When nerve or muscle damage is suspected, special testing can be done to determine the degree of damage and if the damage is specifically to the nerve or muscle. There are two tests that are most commonly used for this purpose.

EMG or *electromyography* is a test in which a tiny fine wire is inserted into a particular muscle. This wire is attached to a machine that records the electrical activity of the muscle. Normal muscle at rest presents a specific pattern of electrical impulse. If the muscle is damaged or paralyzed, it will present a different type of pattern of activity. The activity is recorded on a TV-like screen and is also traced on paper as a graph. If the muscle is not getting enough nerve stimulation, the amplitude of the activity is diminished. If too much stimulation occurs, such as in a spastic muscle, the amplitude will be higher than normal. Therefore, if there is doubt about muscle function or activity, an EMG can be helpful in diagnosis.

Nerve-conduction tests measure the rate an impulse travels down a nerve to make a muscle contract or twitch. If the nerve being tested is injured, it will take longer for that impulse to travel from the site of stimulation to the muscle involved. In other words, if I stimulate the nerve in your arm that causes your thumb to move, the test will measure the time that it takes from the moment of nerve stimulation to the moment the thumb moves.

These tests are generally done in a doctor's office, either by a nurse, neurologist, or a physiatrist. They are not performed routinely, only when there is doubt as to the diagnosis or which muscles or nerves are involved. When muscle weakness is due to a herniated disk, and it is obvious on examination, these tests are not indicated. However, if symptoms are vague and normal muscle testing is inconclusive, then these tests are very helpful in determining muscle abnormalities and which nerve roots may be involved.

If you have been reading along without a break, it is time to take a seventh-inning stretch. I have filled your mind with all sorts of facts and ideas about back pain and leg pain, what causes these pains, and even how to diagnose the causes. You are even conversant with the most up-to-date sophisticated tests that are used in making a diagnosis. You are also aware that I believe most back problems can be helped with a program of low-back exercises and also general-body exercises. Before I get into the exercise section, I shall describe the multitudinous types of treatment that are offered to back-pain sufferers: from chiropractor to acupuncture, from physical therapy to surgery. So now is the time to take that stretch, get the blood flowing, and then resume your reading and learning (I hope) about treatment for back pain.

TREATMENT

Now that the tests are completed and a diagnosis of your problem has been reached, it is time to move on to the treatments that will provide you with relief from pain, currently and in the future. It is time to emphasize, once again, that despite the variety of sophisticated medical and surgical procedures, which I shall be describing shortly, in the final analysis it is *you and only you* who can ensure the long term success of the treatments.

Manipulative Treatment

Chiropractors and osteopaths attempt to manipulate away back pain. They are often successful, especially if the problem is related to a facet joint or muscle spasm. On the other hand, the treatment of a herniated disk by manipulation is not very successful. Remember, 90 percent of all patients with back pain eventually get better regardless of the treatment, or in fact if they have no treatment, so that relieving the present pain is only a temporary solution to the problem. The key to the permanent solution is that once the pain is gone, patients must do back exercises and do them for the rest of their lives. Recently I have been very pleased to see that chiropractors and osteopaths are advising their patients to do back exercises once their pain is relieved. That is good judgment and good treatment for the patient.

There are a few misconceptions about manipulation that I would like to dispel. The first is that manipulation "can slip the herniated disk back into place." That is physically impossible. Manipulation can reduce facet impingement and relieve muscle spasm, but once a disk has slipped out, herniated through the ligament, it cannot be reinserted between the vertebral bodies. It remains out unless surgically removed or chemically dissolved.

Another misconception is that manipulation corrects leg-length discrepancy. Actually, when your back is in spasm, you are twisted, and you walk as though one leg were shorter. If the manipulation is successful in relaxing the spasm, the spine straightens, and the leg no longer appears short! The manipulation has not corrected a basic malalignment or anatomic anomaly of the spine. If the manipulation relieves spasm, it allows the spine to resume its normal alignment. In so doing, mobility is restored to the spine, and that is very helpful.

Osteopaths are also skilled in the manipulation of the body. Unlike chiropractors, they have attended a four-year osteopathic medical school that has the same curriculum and courses as most medical schools. They are licensed to practice medicine, like M.D.'s, but also have manipulative skills. Some osteopaths go on to specialty training and become surgeons.

Acupuncture and Local Injections

I cannot explain why acupuncture works, but it has relieved pain in some cases. Many of my patients have undergone acupuncture treatments. Very few of them have had any significant short-term or long-term benefits from these treatments. However, since bad side effects are rare, I do not object to my patient who is having a difficult time with pain trying to find relief with acupuncture. I know several fine acupuncturists in New York City to whom I refer patients. If they think that acupuncture can be helpful, they will treat the patient; otherwise they will not attempt this treatment. Once in a while patients have responded well to acupuncture when all else has been of no avail.

Many doctors provide local injection treatments for low-back pain. These injections into muscles or ligaments consist of plain saline solutions, local anesthetics alone, or local anesthetics mixed with a cortisone preparation. The injections, which are generally given in the doctor's office, are for relief of muscle inflammation, an inflamed joint, or for a *fibromyositis*. In general, the doctor will carefully press along the spine or pelvic region until he finds a tender spot. He will then inject this tender spot with the medication. Injections are inconsistent in relieving localized spasm, and if successful, provide only temporary relief and in no way solve the problem.

EPIDURAL INJECTIONS

Whereas I might be skeptical about the benefits of local injections and acupuncture, I prescribe with greater confidence epidural cortisone and facet injections. These injections under controlled conditions are given directly into the "root" (pardon the pun) of the problem to relieve pain. Epidural injections have been used by anesthesiologists for many years to anesthetize the pelvic area and the legs. They are similar to spinal anesthesia, except that the anesthetic agent is placed outside the cord membrane rather than inside (the preface *epi* means outside the dura, which is the lining membrane of the spinal cord). It is safer than spinal anesthesia and is less likely to cause subsequent headaches or nausea.

In our hospital, these injections are given by the anesthesiologists who have the most experience with this type of injection. When I refer the patient to the anesthesiologist, I also provide information regarding the diagnosis and location of the problem. If X-rays, CT scan, or MRI are available, I will send them along for review.

The anesthesiologist injects the appropriate area with a cortisone preparation and a small amount of local anesthesia. Nerve roots are bathed in the solution, relieving irritation and inflammation. Patients with disk herniations and nerve problems or with spinal stenosis are often helped by these injections. Unfortunately the relief may only be temporary, necessitating further injections or other treatment.

FACET INJECTIONS

These injections require X-ray control. The doctor, usually a radiologist (but many other specialists are qualified) places a needle right at the facet joint and confirms this placement with X-rays. An injection of cortisone and a local anesthetic is then given into the facet-joint region. If the facet joint is inflamed and the cause of discomfort, the pain is relieved. Often patients with facet-joint problems develop inflammation of the underlying nerve root, so that the pain radiates into the leg, simulating typical sciatica. When treatment is successful, pain from the joint and its radiating component will subside. The relief may only be temporary, lasting a few days to a few months, but the injections can be repeated if necessary.

Other Forms of Treatment:
Heat, Cold, Deep Massage, Ultrasound, Diathermy, and Electrical Stimulation

I lump all of these methods of treatment together because they are similar in that they are *modalities*. A modality is something that is applied to the surface of the body that is expected to have a beneficial effect on the deep structures that need treatment. These methods are not curative, but do provide temporary relief and perhaps will help speed the rate of recovery.

In regard to heat and cold, I recommend application of ice to the lower back in an acute injury or in the initial stages of pain. It should be applied for twenty minutes at a time. The ice itself should be wrapped in a towel so that it is not directly against the skin. I have seen patients with "ice burns" on their backs when ice has been applied directly against the skin and left on too long. For chronic nagging backaches, not severe, a heating pad or hot-water bottle is soothing. Moist heat generally provides more comfort than dry heat. Be careful never to use anything too hot against the skin because of potential burns. Unmindful use of heating pads and hydrocolators can result in very bad burns.

Massage and rolfing (deep, hard massage) are low on my list for treatment. They do provide beneficial relaxation and make you feel good, but do not really affect the cause of your pain. Anyone who can tolerate rolfing massage should be able to tolerate most back pain. A patient returned to me with large bruises all over her body from a rolfing session. Yet she said that it helped her. For all she went through, I hope it did.

Ultrasound and diathermy are methods used to penetrate deep into the tissues of the spine to deliver heat that supposedly has a healing affect. Ultrasound obviously does this by sending sound waves into the deep tissues, and diathermy by projecting heat into the deeper muscles. Many physical therapists employ these techniques to "loosen up" the back before treatment. If used in that way, then modalities are purposeful, but if used as the only method of treatment by themselves, they have very little merit.

Medications

Patients often ask for the magic pill that can cure their pain. It would be wonderful if such a medication existed. "Here, take this pill, it will cure your back problem." Unfortunately such a pill does not exist. There is no quick fix for back sufferers. However, medications do have a significant role to play in the treatment of aching backs and legs. Three types of medicines are helpful—muscle relaxants, anti-inflammatories, and analgesics.

Muscle relaxants are those substances that loosen up or relax tight or spastic muscles. Most of the time these substances produce muscle relaxation by exerting a tranquilizing effect upon the brain. As yet, a muscle relaxant that works directly upon the muscle without affecting the brain has not been produced. Most of the common muscle relaxants—Norflex, Robaxin, Soma, and Flexeril—are all examples of muscle relaxants whose primary effect is central, that is, on the basic nervous system and brain rather than directly on the muscle. Valium (diazepam), the well-known tranquilizer, is also a muscle relaxant, but should be used very cautiously because of its addictive tendency. It is the tranquilizing property of the medication that leads to the muscle relaxation that is helpful in the acute phase of back and sciatic attacks.

Anti-inflammatory medications reduce inflammation in the muscles, joints, and ligaments of the spine. Cortisone and cortisone preparations are the strongest anti-inflammatory drugs, but because of potential side effects, are used only sparingly. In the past several years, a large number of noncortisone anti-inflammatory agents have been developed. These include the ibuprofen group, such as Motrin, Advil, Nuprin, etc., and a dozen other different preparations, such as indomethacin (Indocin), Naprosyn, Clinoril, Feldene, and Voltaren, etc.

These are all given to reduce inflammation and pain in the spine and adjoining areas. These medications may be used for a short term, such as one or two weeks, or in some instances patients may be kept on these medications for many months. The ability of a medication to relieve pain varies greatly among people. In some individuals, one anti-inflammatory medicine may be very helpful, whereas in someone else, the same drug may not be effective. One common problem with all of the anti-inflammatory medications is that they can produce irritation of the stomach and intestines. This can result in nausea, heartburn, stomachache, vomiting, diarrhea, and even may cause ulcers that can bleed. I do not mean to scare you. I prescribe these medications every day, but I caution my patients to stop the medication immediately if any of these symptoms appear. I ask that they call me right away so that I can record the adverse affect. Muscle relaxants and anti-inflammatory medications can be safely given together.

Analgesics are the other frequently prescribed medication for painful backs. These compounds do not treat the cause of the pain, but only relieve the pain itself. Tylenol and aspirin compounds may be ineffective in relieving pain associated with back syndromes. Usually prescription medication containing codeine or codeinelike substances, such as Percodan, Tylenol with codeine, Vicodin, aspirin with codeine, etc., are necessary. Their pain-relieving ability is generally quite good. Codeine and its derivatives are narcotics, and can be habit-forming. These drugs should be used carefully and sparingly. Stronger narcotics that are given by injection, such as Demerol and morphine, are prescribed only in a hospital setting and given for the most severe pains.

Before leaving the topic of medications, I want to emphasize that pain relievers are rarely necessary for more than two or three days. Even individuals with severe back spasm and leg pain from a herniated disk can obtain relief from pain by sufficient bed rest. Finding the most comfortable position in bed is essential. Lying on the side with one or both knees curled up, the so-called fetal position, relieves the pain for most people. Also, it is important in the acute phase of pain to stay in bed continuously. Every time you get up to have a meal or go to the bathroom, you are re-irritating your back and delaying your recovery. The first forty-eight hours are of particular importance. During this time, the more consistent the bed rest, the less stress and strain on your back, and the more rapidly your back symptoms will subside.

So far I have described what can be done to indirectly help your back—that is, to relieve inflammation and pain—but not really to correct the source of the pain, which is usually an unstable back with or without a herniated disk. Exercises, if carried out daily, can control pain in 80 to 90 percent of all back problems. For the others who are not conscientious enough in their exercise program, or whose condition is too unstable, or whose disk is too herniated, direct-intervention therapy is required. That means either dissolving the disk with an enzyme or surgery for removal of the disk. Surgery will also be required for relief of spinal stenosis and for fusion of the spine when it is necessary to obtain stability. Without going into "gory" details, I shall briefly describe what each of these procedures entails.

Dissolving the Disk: Chemonucleosis

The nucleus pulposus, the soft central portion of the disk, which is the actual substance that protrudes or herniates, consists of a protein material (collagen) and water. Chymopapain, an enzyme derived from papaya, can be injected into the disk to dissolve the nucleus pulposus. The procedure is done with the patient awake and with X-ray control. A needle is inserted in the back, into the intervertebral disk space. When X-rays ascertain that the needle is in the midportion of the disk space, a small amount of the enzyme is injected. At the time of the injection, the patient may feel pain in the leg similar to the radiating type of pain he or she has been experiencing. Otherwise, the procedure is relatively painless. Hospitalization following the procedure is usually recommended for one or two days, and then the patient can return to light work but must be careful in activities for approximately six weeks.

The disadvantages of this method are that some people are allergic to the papaya enzyme and can develop a severe reaction, and that if the enzyme comes in contact with the nerve root itself, it can inflame and irritate the nerve. Over the years, there has been a marked decrease in the use of chemonucleosis, partly because of the complications, but also because there were a large number of patients in whom the pain was not relieved. The indications for this enzyme injection are now fairly well limited to those patients who have not had disk surgery at the same level, have failed conservative treatment, are not pregnant, and have no history of an allergy to papaya or other significant allergies. In addition, the disk itself should still be contained within the annulus fibrosis— that is, not completely extruded into the spinal canal. Patients with significant abnormal neurological findings usually have completely herniated disks and are not good candidates for this procedure. Older patients with arthritis and spinal stenosis are also not good candidates for chymopapain injections. In these patients, nerve-root compression is caused by other factors that are not relieved by simply dissolving the disk.

Percutaneous Aspiration of the Disk

Percutaneous removal of a disk is a relatively new procedure. It consists of placing a large hollow needle into the disk space and sucking out the disk material or removing it with a rotary reamer device. Enzymes are not injected with this procedure so that there is no risk of an allergic reaction or nerve damage, which may accompany the chemonucleosis procedure. However, this procedure has several significant limitations. First, the long-term effects of removing the disk in this fashion are unknown. Second, only the material inside the disk space can be removed, leaving pieces of disk in the spinal canal that can cause problems. Third, the L5–S1 disk space is often difficult to enter because of the overlapping pelvic bones, and almost half of all herniations occur in this disk space. Finally, if there is pressure on the nerve root from a small canal (stenosis) or thickening of the overlying ligaments, pressures caused by these structures cannot be removed by percutaneous extraction of the disk. Nevertheless, in selective cases, percutaneous aspiration of the disk may be successful.

Surgical Removal of the Herniated Disk

Since Mixter and Barr in 1934 publicized their article on the relief of sciatica with removal of a herniated disk, this procedure has been used worldwide to treat patients with slipped disks. Over the years, the surgical technique has been refined with improvement in the overall results. It has become increasingly clear that herniation of the disk alone is only part of the problem causing the pain: a narrow canal, thickened ligaments, and bony spurs all play a role in irritating and compressing the involved nerve root. Thus, the operation no longer means just removing the protruding disk, but also includes decompressing and removing any pressure on the nerve root.

The standard procedure is to make an incision over the involved disk space. The muscles are retracted from the spinal bones so that the space between the adjoining vertebral bodies can be seen. A ligament lies between those two bones and is removed. The space is made wider by cutting off small pieces of the bone on either side of the space. This exposes the dural sac and nerve root. The herniated portion of the disk can be seen by moving aside the nerve root and the dural sac. The extruded disk is now removed. Any bony spurs or edges of bone that press or compromise the passage of the nerve root are also removed. If fragments of the disk remain inside the disk space, these are removed as well. Obviously, during this procedure, the nerve root and dural sac are carefully protected.

Microdiscectomy is a variation of the standard procedure in which a microscope or a magnifying lens is used to help visualize the disk and remove it. The procedure is done through a small incision, and the scope and instruments are placed through this incision. The advantage of this method is that hospitalization is shorter and the patient has a quicker return to all activities, including work. However, the operation takes longer when a microscope is used, and because of the limited exposure of the area, there is greater potential to miss fragments of an extruded disk. It is also more difficult to thoroughly decompress the nerve root with this smaller exposure.

Decompression for Spinal Stenosis

The patient with spinal stenosis has narrowing of the spinal canal, which causes pressure on the nerve roots. This may be associated with disk degeneration or herniation. In order to relieve this pressure, the spinal canal must be enlarged. This procedure unroofs the spinal canal and removes all pressure from the nerve roots. If a disk herniation is involved, it too can be removed. Lateral spinal stenosis is caused by spurs that form under the facet joints. These spurs become large enough to compress the underlying nerve root and must be excised in order to relieve the pressure on the roots. Occasionally the small canal (foramen) through which the nerve root exits from the spinal canal is also constricted and can cause compression of the nerve root. This canal too must be enlarged if relief of symptoms is to be obtained. Enlarging this canal is known as *foraminotomy*.

In summary, the treatment of spinal stenosis involves enlarging the spinal canal, removing herniated-disk fragments, excising bony spurs from the facet joints, and performing a foraminotomy when necessary. This can be a complex operation, and furthermore, it usually involves more than one segment of the spine. Many patients have this operation performed from L1 to the sacrum. As noted, spinal stenosis is much more frequent in people of sixty years and older, many of whom have significant medical problems, which can further complicate the surgery.

Fortunately anesthetic procedures have vastly improved in the past ten to fifteen years. Patients can be monitored extremely closely, and complications of anesthesia are now infrequent. The advances made in anesthesiology have allowed surgeons in all fields to perform much more complex and lengthy operations than ever before. As a surgeon, I am acutely aware of what is happening at the head of the operating table. Good anesthesia techniques mean that my efforts on the table will be well sustained to ensure a successful result for the patient. I take this opportunity to publicly express my admiration and respect for the expert anesthesiologists who work with me at the Hospital for Special Surgery. I have the pleasure and peace of mind of working with an excellent group of doctors.

Spine Fusion

Eventually most back sufferers hear the term *spine fusion*. Often it is said with a sense of dread or foreboding. "Poor guy, he had a spine fusion," or "She had a fusion eight months ago and still can't walk." What is a spine fusion, and why do back patients have that operation? The "what" should be explained first. A vertebral bone is a separate entity, and if I were to cut all the attaching ligaments and muscles, I could separate each bone from the other. The ligaments and intervertebral disk hold the bones together, but also allow motion between the adjacent bones, which is why the spine is flexible. Motion in the thoracic spine is limited by the attachment of the ribs, whereas the lumbar spine has no rib attachments and thus a greater range of motion.

If there is damage to an intervertebral disk and to the facet joints, the movements of one vertebral bone on the other may be abnormal. This instability can be quite painful. Most often it occurs in the lower-lumbar spine—i.e., between L4 and L5 and L5 and S1. Spondylolysis and spondylolisthesis can result in abnormal movement and pain. Patients who have had extensive laminectomies for spinal stenosis may also have instability with abnormal movement.

Braces for the back are often used to try to "stabilize" the lower back and prevent this abnormal motion. Unfortunately braces are frequently ineffective in controlling this situation. If an external brace does not help, what about an internal brace to hold the bones together? Such a brace would prevent motion between the two bones, thereby eliminating pain. Well, that is what a spine fusion accomplishes; it holds the two adjoining vertebral bones together so that motion cannot occur. It is done with bone chips and becomes a permanent bonding.

Most people are aware that if a bone breaks and the ends are held together in a cast, the bone ends will grow together and heal. In spine fusion, slivers or chips taken from the pelvic bone are grafted to fuse with the adjoining vertebra to form a solid mass. Once the fusion is solid, no motion can occur between the two bones. Occasionally more than two vertebrae are fused together. The L5 is most often fused to the S1 vertebra, but sometimes L4 and even L3 have to be added to the fusion.

Patients with scoliosis may need a spine fusion from the upper thoracic spine down to the lower-lumbar spine, but that operation, although still a fusion, is done for very different reasons than the fusions for low-back problems.

There are various techniques for performing the fusion. It can be done entirely from the back of the spine, or the side of the spine, but rarely from the front of the spine. This latter method necessitates going through the abdomen and is a much more complicated procedure.

In recent years, in order to help stabilize the spine while the bone slivers are healing to the vertebral bodies, some orthopedic surgeons have been using screws and metal plates on the bones to prevent motion. Most straightforward spine fusions are successful without the use of metal fixations. However, in complicated cases, the use of screws and plates can be of significant help in obtaining a solid fusion.

An amazing aspect of a spine fusion is that although it eliminates motion between one or more vertebral bones, the patient is not really aware of the functional loss of motion. Bending from the hips is still possible, and the remaining vertebral joints retain some movement.

In the early days of excision of herniated intervertebral disks, fusion of the two involved vertebrae was done almost routinely. Orhopedic surgeons at the time believed that because the disk structure was no longer intact, abnormal motions would occur and eventually lead to pain. Over the years, that theory has proven to be incorrect. Unless extensive laminectomy and removal of the facet joints are done at the same time as the disk excision, instability does not occur. Today, it is very rare to perform a spine fusion in conjunction with removal of a disk. However, not all disks are excised under the same conditions, so occasionally a fusion may be necessary. Another reason why fusions are not done routinely is that a fusion is a very extensive procedure, and it takes several months before the patient is able to return to normal activities, compared to several weeks for someone who has had a standard disk excision.

Failed Back Surgery

Although the results of disk surgery and spinal fusions are generally successful in 80 to 90 percent of the patients, there are some patients who continue to have pain after surgery. The reason for post-surgical pain varies. Scarring of nerve roots, excess spurring, retained disk fragments, disk herniations at more than one level, and instability between two vertebral bones are all possible causes of persistent pain. Determining the exact cause of pain after surgery is difficult. Usually CT and MRI scans need to be performed, and often a myelogram may be necessary.

When surgery does not eliminate the pain, it is important to proceed cautiously and slowly with the patient. Patience by the patient and doctor alike is necessary. A strict program of rest, exercise, and medication over time can often result in relief of symptoms, thus permitting a return to normal activities. If further testing reveals that the continued pain can be relieved by another operation, then additional surgery may resolve the problem. However, unless the diagnosis is very specific, it is better not to operate again. An "exploratory" back operation is not usually successful, and often leaves the patient worse than before.

Because back surgery is not always successful, it must be approached with great caution. About 80 percent of the patients with disk problems will get better with time and rest. I strongly believe that if these patients are taught to care for their backs properly and to perform regular daily back exercises, they will never require surgery for their slipped disks. However, for that remaining small group whose disk herniations cause unrelenting pain or muscle weakness, surgery is necessary, and as noted, is successful in 80 to 90 percent of the cases.

Bear in mind that surgery for removal of a herniated disk or even for a spine fusion is only part of the solution for a back problem. Remember that after a herniated disk is removed, the integrity of the structure consisting of the disk and the two adjoining vertebrae and the facets has been permanently damaged. In order to prevent future problems as the result of this basic damage to the joint, the weakened area has to be protected and strengthened by proper body mechanics, which means practicing proper methods of lifting, sitting, and carrying to reduce excessive stress on the weakened area. It is strengthened by firming the muscles that support the lower spine—the back, stomach, and hip muscles. Improvement in body mechanics is also gained by removing any tight or contracted forces about the spine: If hamstrings are tight, they should be stretched; if hip flexors are contracted, they should be stretched; if there is an excessive lordosis, this should be corrected.

A combination, then, of good body mechanics and strong muscles of the spine is essential for a healthy back and "no more aching back." Even after an operation, recurrent problems can only be prevented by a good exercise program, which only you can do. An unhappy experience is for back-surgery patients to have initial good results, only to be followed by recurrence of pain. One of the major reasons for this is that these patients do not persist with their exercise program. They do their "physical therapy" until they are feeling well, and then gradually they stop exercising. At first they may feel no ill effects from lack of exercise, but eventually they will be doomed to recurring problems with their backs.

I stress the importance of an exercise program at the end of this section on treatment. In a sense, all of the treatments that I have so far described treat the end result of a back problem—that is, the end result of a mechanical instability of the back. However, to treat the origin of the symptoms, an exercise program is essential.

5. Everyday Living and Your Back

Throughout this book, I refer to the proper way to use your back and make suggestions as to how that goal can be achieved. I thought it might be helpful if I collected all those hints and recommendations into one chapter and made them easily available for your review. I shall separate this section into three parts, and relate each part to your body's posture or position.

LYING DOWN

What is so important about the way we lie down? It is a simple enough position; gravity is relieved, and your back rests. Well, how and on what you sleep is important to your back's health. First, start with the mattress. (See Figure 14.) A poor mattress allows your back to sag and can cause additional back stress. A good mattress should be firm, but not necessarily "rock hard." A platform bed provides good support for the spine. A bed board (three-quarter-inch plywood is fine) placed under a soft mattress also provides adequate support for your back. Always test a new mattress before you buy it. Sit on the edge. Determine how much it sags or gives way to your body weight.

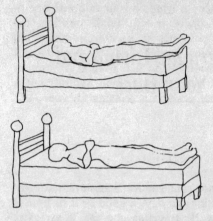

SAGGING MATTRESS

FIRM MATTRESS

Mattresses with minimal sag are best. I do not recommend any specific mattress. All the better companies have firm or orthopedic-type mattresses. Just try them yourself. Older people or individuals with arthritis or other infirmities may find a hard mattress extremely uncomfortable. If this is the case, adding a two-inch foam-rubber pad on top of the mattress can ease the pressure on bony prominences when you're lying down and make you much more comfortable.

The position in which you lie is also important. Many people like to sleep on their stomachs and can do so without pain or discomfort. However, once you have developed a back problem, particularly a slipped disk, this position is often uncomfortable and even painful. On the other hand, lying flat on your back can also be painful. If you have back problems and want to sleep on your back, place two or three pillows under your knees so that your hips and knees are bent. I am certain that you will find this to be a comfortable position. However, the overall best position in which to sleep is lying on your side with one or both knees bent—the so-called "fetal" position, the way in which the baby lies in the uterus—curled up, with the thighs against the chest and the heels against the buttocks. Obviously the actual fetal position is extreme and one that would not be natural, but a modification of that position is relaxing for your back and thus for you.

SITTING

Most people do not spend more than seven to eight hours in bed. During the day, a good deal of time is spent sitting—at work, traveling in a car, in a movie, watching TV, or in a classroom. We sit because it is easier than standing. In fact, when we sit, the muscles in our back and stomach relax. Because of this relaxation, it is vital that we sit with our bodies in good alignment; otherwise the stress on the intervertebral disks, ligaments, and facet joints can be excessive. The type of chair on which you sit deserves a great deal of consideration. Back-pain sufferers avoid soft easy chairs like the plague. They have learned by bitter experience that if they sit in a soft easy chair or couch for an extended time, they will have stiffness and pain in their back when they arise. When they go into someone else's home, you will see them scan the room for a solid chair before they sit down. The soft easy chair allows the spine to sag, usually reversing the lumbar lordosis, and that position is strenuous for the back. Choose a good firm chair; those with a thin cushion are satisfactory. You should be able to sit with the small of your back against the back of the chair. With your knees bent at a 90-degree angle, both feet should rest comfortably on the floor. (See Figure 15.) Chairs with arms are preferable because they help when you get up. Swivel chairs are also acceptable as long as the seat and back are fixed. Chairs in which the back extends separately from the seat portion are a potential source of low-back problems. Check your chairs at home and at work to make certain that they fit you comfortably.

The "teenage slouch" is such a characteristic posture that just mentioning the word brings to mind a sixteen-year-old who is stretched out on a chair with head and neck resting on the top of the chair and buttocks on the edge of the seat. The legs are straight, and the heels rest on the floor. The spine has no contact with the chair and is suspended in midair from the neck to the buttocks. While a teenager can survive this position, I fear for you and me. We would be in a real fix after an hour or so. As noted, you should sit fairly straight and upright in the chair, your lower back against the back of the chair and your feet resting comfortably on the floor.

SITTING POSTURE #15

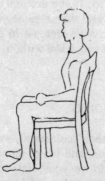 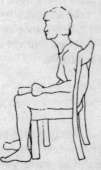

GOOD SITTING POSTURE   POOR SITTING POSTURE

When you drive a car, the same rules apply. Sit closer to the wheel so that your hips and knees are flexed. Do not drive with your legs stretched out in front of you, because that puts a strain on your lower back. If your seat is adjustable, then tilt the seat back 10 or 15 degrees so that instead of being straight up, you incline very slightly backward. This position rests your back. For individuals in whom the lumbar lordosis is relatively fixed, the use of a small pad or pillow in the lumbar region of a car seat or a chair can also provide additional comfort, especially for prolonged sitting or driving.

While we are discussing driving, *never*, and I mean *never*, while sitting in the front seat of the car, twist around to pick up something from the floor or seat behind you. That twisting and lifting motion can be disastrous for your back, as illustrated by the case history of Mr. R.

If you have had serious back problems in the past or have recently recovered from a "back attack," avoid sitting for lengthy periods. After one hour, stand up and walk around. Stretch a little and then sit down again. If you are in an airplane, walk up and down the aisle at least every hour or so. If you are in a car, stop the car, take a short stroll, and then resume your trip. If you are at a movie or in a theater, sit in the back row so that you can get up and stand without disturbing other people.

STANDING

People do many things on their feet: stand, walk, run, lift, carry objects, play sports, and jump, among other activities. The more you do on your feet, the more you have to be concerned about your back.

The primary consideration when standing is your posture. Proper posture is the head balanced over the spine and pelvis. Good posture starts with control of the pelvis, avoiding excess lumbar lordosis, and holding the head high (not the chin), so that the shoulders will naturally come erect. (See Figure 16.) Good posture should feel comfortable but does require constant effort, both physical and mental. It takes practice to maintain good posture and walk, but after a while it becomes second nature.

In addition to good posture, good shoe wear is important for walking. Women may feel that they look better in high heels, but those extra inches on the heel cause an accentuation of lumbar lordosis that is not good for the back. Fortunately most women wear high heels only for special occasions and not for long walks or exercise. For women and men, comfortable, well-fitting shoes that are not tight are essential for comfortable walking and also help the back. Usually a lace shoe fits better and provides more support for the foot.

STANDING POSTURE #16

GOOD POSTURE   POOR POSTURE

Most lifting and bending activities are done while standing, so I shall discuss how these are done in this section. Probably the most important advice I can give you in this regard is never to twist your back and lift, and never to lift and twist your back. In other words, if you are about to pick up a box (or even your shoes), square off your body and shoulders so that you face the box, then bend your knees and bend forward. There is no need to keep your back rigid and do a knee bend. If you bend your knees first, you can lean forward without stressing your lower back. If you are picking up something heavy, place one foot in front of the other (with your feet somewhat apart), bend your knees, lean forward, and then lift the object to your body. (See Figure 17.) Once you have it securely in your grasp, straighten your legs; let them do the work, not your back. If the box you lifted has to be placed on a table, turn to face the table with your feet, do not twist your trunk, and then place the box down. The reverse is also true. If you are taking the box from the table and placing it on the floor, lift the box to your body, turn to where you want to place the box, put one foot in front of the other, bend your knees, and then bend your upper body toward the floor to place the box where you want it.

Be careful not to lift something that is too heavy for you. Either get someone to help or lighten the load amd make two trips.

Another source of danger is lifting above your shoulders. If you extend your arms straight out in front of you and gradually lift them over your head, you will notice that as you elevate your arms, your back arches; that is a natural phenomenon. However, if you perform the same maneuver with a heavy weight in your hands, you are causing great strain on your lower back. Lifting a heavy box of books and trying to place

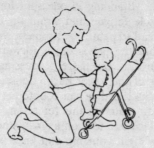

it on a high shelf in the closet could be a catastrophic event for you. The stress that this places on your lower back could easily rupture a disk. Get a stool or solid chair, put the books on an easily accessible height, and then lift and put them on the shelf. Lifting above your shoulders is dangerous not only with heavy objects but light ones as well. So when you have to place a pile of dishes into a kitchen cabinet, stand on a stool to do so. Spare your back. Remember, in order to avoid problems with your back, you have to use your head as well as your muscles.

Bending over is not without its consequences. Women tend to be more supple or limber than men. Many women, without any special stretching or exercise activity, can easily touch the floor with their knees straight. It becomes a natural habit for them to bend over in that fashion at all times: knees locked straight and bending over from the lower spine. This is dangerous, because one day you may bend over and not be able to straighten up. Whenever you bend, whether to open the oven and check on the roast, or to scratch the cat's ear, bend your knees first. (See Figure 18.) *There are absolutely no exceptions to this rule, and I cannot be emphatic enough.*

Many people complain that just standing is painful for their backs. Standing in one spot for a long time increases muscle fatigue and strain on the back and does indeed lead to pain. The problem with prolonged standing is that the pelvis drops forward, increasing the lumbar lordosis and thereby stressing the muscles and ligaments of the lower back. Consciously clenching the buttocks together can counteract the standing lordosis, but to maintain this for a long time is difficult. If you place one foot on a small stool or footrest several inches high, your hip and knee will bend and the pelvis is shifted backward, reducing the lordois. When I operate for long hours, I have a footstool handy so that I can rest upon it. If the procedure is particularly long, I shift from foot to foot. This prevents fatigue and back pain, and not only allows me to stand and operate for many hours, but also prevents me from having an aching back after the surgery is completed.

Similarly it is wise to use a small footrest when

BENDING OVER #18

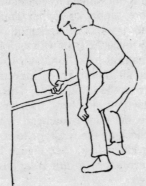

ironing or during other standing activities. Bars and taverns often have a rail on which the drinker rests his foot. Tavern owners have learned that if you can stand comfortably for more hours, you will also be able to drink more.

Carrying objects can also be hazardous for someone with back problems. I am often asked the question, "How much can I lift and carry?" My answer is that the amount you carry is not the crux of the problem, it is how you carry the weight, although an individual's size is a factor. A 250-pound football player can carry 100 pounds easily. A 125-pound female should not even consider carrying that much weight. However, regardless of the amount of weight you are about to carry, you must always carry it properly.

Carrying large, bulky items is more difficult than carrying compact items even if the compact item weighs more. The problem with bulky items is that your arms are just not long enough to get around them. It makes the carrying very difficult and places an excessive load on your back. The wise course to follow is to have someone help you carry that bulky package, whether it weighs thirty pounds or one hundred pounds. Compact weights like a box of books may be very heavy, but if you lift them properly, hold them close to your chest, and do not carry them too far, your back is probably safe.

Third World natives (among others) often carry heavy objects on their heads, and do so without hurting their spines. The key to carrying this weight is balance. With the weight balanced on the head, the shoulders, spine, and pelvis are kept in perfect alignment so that the weight is evenly distributed down the spine to the legs. If you have practiced this method of carrying from childhood, you should be able to continue to do so without difficulty. But if you have not, I would not recommend that you try now.

Holding boxes on your shoulder is a comfortable and less strenuous method of carrying heavy weights. Your ability to do this depends upon your own strength and the weight to be carried. When I have to carry a heavy box for a long distance, I find that changing the position in which I hold the box prevents fatigue and excess strain. I shift the box from shoulder to shoulder and sometimes carry it against my chest. Changing carrying positions diminishes fatigue and strain.

Time and again in the history of man, we discover that things we thought were new and modern were actually part of the daily lives of people centuries ago. Certainly that applies to carrying heavy objects on one's back. Today, the backpacker frees his hands and lets his back do the carrying. When I was a child, I carried my books to school under my arm or in a briefcase. My children had backpacks in which to put their books and carry them. Carrying the weight in a backpack is similar to carrying a weight on the head. The weight exerts a downward pressure, which is taken up by the shoulder straps and evenly distributed down the spine to the legs.

Because scoliosis (a sideways curve of the back) is seen predominantly in girls from ten to fourteen years of age, it was thought to result from carrying a bookbag on one shoulder; the weight twisted the body to one side, resulting in scoliosis. This theory was repudiated many years ago, but it is much healthier for the back if the weight is evenly distributed rather than unevenly placed on one side. Indeed, next time you have to carry a heavy package of groceries home from the store, have the grocer make two equally weighted packages. The balanced weights prevent uneven stress on your back. The same principle applies to traveling.

For some reason, people always tend to travel with one bag. It is usually a big bag and tightly packed. Lifting a heavy bag is bad enough, but to carry it on one side is a disaster! Be sensible; pack two bags instead of one, or even three instead of two. The bags will be easier to lift and safer to carry.

6. Back Pain in Children

Back problems in children are different from those in adults. These differences are significant enough to merit a special section in this book. I shall define a child as someone who is still growing, and generally under sixteen years of age.

The growth factor is extremely important, because as the bone grows longer (in the case of the vertebral bones, higher), the muscles and ligaments that are attached to the bones elongate. The ligaments in children are very strong and are actually stronger than the bones that they connect. When a child sustains an injury to his or her knee, the bone will break before the ligament tears. Often in children, if forces are sufficient, rather than the ligament tearing, it will pull off a piece of bone, resulting in an *avulsion fracture*. This type of fracture occurs in the knees and ankles of children.

The same disparity between the strength of the ligament and bones exists in the spine of the child. Earlier in this book, I described the conditions of *spondylolysis* and *spondylolisthesis*. I stated that these conditions are more common in children than adults, and in fact probably occurred in childhood and persisted in adult life. Both of these conditions are due to physical stress on a specific area of the vertebral bone, the pars interarticularis. Because the supporting ligaments are very strong, when specific forces are maintained over a long period of time, it is the bone that gives way, not the ligament. As noted in young athletes, particularly young girls who are avid gymnasts, their strenuous and excessive spinal movements can cause an acute fracture of the pars interarticularis.

The symptoms of an acute fracture are obvious. The child complains of pain in his or her back. The spine is held stiffly and often tilted to one side. The pain is localized to the back without leg radiation. A history of injury or strain is always present. The actual injury may have occurred several hours or even a day or two before the child begins complaining of pain.

Physical examination will reveal local muscle spasm in the spine and limited motions. Tenderness to pressure over the injured area is also present. X-rays are necessary to make the diagnosis. In some instances, a bone scan is necessary to localize the site of the fracture. Treatment is straightforward—a back brace for six to eight weeks results in healing of the fracture. After the fracture is healed and the brace eliminated, I would recommend a program of back exercises for these children.

The chronic type of spondylolysis has less obvious symptoms. The child complains of intermittent back pain that is not well localized. Activities aggravate the pain, and rest generally relieves it. Examination may be normal, or may reveal mild limitations of movements of the lower back. If the symptoms have been present for several weeks, I would recommend X-rays of the spine.

Children rarely exaggerate their symptoms, especially back symptoms, and if they have significant pain or persistent intermittent pain, a thorough evaluation must be done. The treatment for the chronic type of spondylolysis is the same as that for the acute.

Spondylolisthesis is invariably a chronic problem. That is, it does not result from a single injury, except for violent accidents such as falling from a height or being involved in a car crash. In order for one vertebra, usually the L5, to slide forward on the vertebra below, usually S1, a defect in both pars interarticulari of L5 must exist. If the force persists, the vertebral body slowly slides forward. An injury or sudden strain in the area can cause it to slip further. Not all the slips are progressive. In some patients, X-rays over several years demonstrate that the vertebral body does not move any further. However, in others the slip is progressive.

Symptoms of spondylolisthesis are similar to those of spondylolysis. Back pain is common, often associated with muscle spasm, stiffness, and listing to one side. When a slip is severe,—that is, if the vertebral bone has slipped almost all the way forward, a step-off of the spinous process can be felt in the lower back.

Whereas a spondylolysis rarely causes sciatic pain in the leg, spondylolisthesis is often associated with radiating leg pain. This sciatica is not caused by a herniated disk, but rather by traction on the nerve roots as the bone slides forward.

The early treatment for spondylolysthesis is immobilization with a back brace. If symptoms disappear and follow-up X-rays reveal that the slip is not progressing, then exercises and avoidance of strenuous athletics are sufficient. If symptoms persist, or if X-rays demonstrate that the slip is progressing, then a fusion operation is necessary. As I previously mentioned, approximately 5 percent of our population have spondylolisthesis. The majority do not require surgery, but all patients with this condition must be followed closely.

Frequently the slip progresses in the younger child. Once growth is complete, the slip usually stabilizes, and surgery is not necessary.

SCOLIOSIS

As mentioned, scoliosis is a problem in young girls that is first observed between the ages of ten and fourteen years. It is rare in boys. The curvature of the spine can be seen by looking at the child's back. (See Figure 7.) It becomes more apparent by having the child bend forward 90 degrees. Scoliosis is not painful in childhood. Occasionally in later adult years, pain from arthritis or pain associated with spinal stenosis may occur. The scoliosis curve may be minimal when first observed and measured on an X-ray. However, as the child grows, the curves get worse. In most cases, after growth has stopped, the curve will not progress. By that time, however, if left untreated, the curve can be very severe, causing a large hump on the young girl's back. If the curve is great enough, the rib cage is compromised, and that can lead to lung and heart problems later in life.

Numerous screening programs to diagnose scoliosis exist throughout the country. Dr. David Levine, one of my colleagues at the Hospital for Special Surgery in New York City, has been a pioneer in the early detection of scoliosis in young girls by routine examinations performed in public school, especially grades seven to ten. As part of a different Pediatric Orthopaedic Outreach Program at our hospital, sponsored by the State of New York, I have examined several hundred younger children in the past two years. Included in the examination is the evaluation of every child's back, regardless of age or sex.

Once a curve is recognized, X-rays of the spine are taken. Mild curves are just observed. Braces are not necessary, and often special back exercises are given to these children. If the curve is moderate, or it if is increasing as documented by serial X-rays, then the child must wear a spinal brace, which usually prevents the curve from getting worse. In order to be effective, the brace must be worn twenty-three out of twenty-four hours. That means the child has to sleep with it on. The brace is worn until growth is complete. If the curve is severe, or progressing despite the brace, then an operation is indicated. The surgery consists of a spine fusion extending over the length of the curve (or curves—frequently there are two) and the use of steel rods to help realign the spine. The results of these operations are very successful, but many children can be successfully treated by braces alone.

Scheurermann's disease affects adolescent males. Don't worry about the name. The disease was named after the doctor who described it. In this condition, the dorsal or thoracic spine curves backward so that the normal kyphosis in this region is markedly increased. This curved posture makes a person very round-shouldered and gives him an appearance of a hunchback. Doctors do not know why it affects boys more than girls (just as we don't know why scoliosis is more prevalent in girls).

When adolescent boys go through a period of rapid growth, three or more dorsal vertebral bodies are compressed along the front of the bones, which causes the curve. These curves can get worse with growth, and they are often associated with pain in the upper back, especially between the shoulder blades. Exercises to strengthen and stretch the upper back are helpful. Some patients require a brace for the upper back to help hold them straighter. In rare cases, surgery is necessary to correct a severe deformity. The mild kyphosis usually is not painful in adult years, but the larger curves can cause pain in later life.

As I mentioned earlier in this chapter, the ligaments in children are stronger than their bones. The combination of strong ligaments and a high water content make disk herniation in children exceedingly rare. I have never seen a child under fifteen with a true disk herniation. I have seen children who have symptoms that mimic disk herniation and sciatica, but after appropriate tests, other causes were found for their pain. Therefore, if a child complains of back pain with radiation of pain to the leg, a disk problem is the least likely cause of the symptoms.

In evaluating children with back and leg pain, the first place to look is in the spine itself. Certain rare types of arthritis can cause pain in children. Small benign tumors of the spine (osteoid osteoma and osteoblastoma) can cause the same symptoms. Infections of the spinal bones can mimic disk problems. Rarely, pain can be caused by calcium deposits in the disks of children.

In other words, a thorough examination and tests are necessary to find out why the child has pain. As I noted, when a child complains of back pain, the pain is real. Children do not exaggerate their symptoms, especially when it comes to the back. Unfortunately adults with back pain often have an emotional aspect to their pain that must be considered in their overall evaluation and treatment.

If the spinal work-up is negative and does not reveal the source of pain, then we have to look elsewhere.

Lyme disease can cause back pain; referred pain from the kidneys or intestinal problems can cause back pain. Blood diseases such as leukemia can be a source of back pain in children as well. The point is that when a child has back pain, with or without sciatic pain, a doctor has to be even better than Sherlock Holmes in uncovering the condition's culprit.

Fortunately back problems are uncommon in children, and most of them can be treated with exercises or braces. However, because some of the conditions that occur in children can be of a serious nature, a thorough evaluation must be performed whenever a child complains of back pain.

7. Sex and the Bad Back

This book would not be complete without dispelling several misconceptions about bad backs and sexual activity. When I was in the early years of my practice, I was somewhat hesitant to discuss questions about sex with my patients. Part of my problem was that although I was a doctor, I was not accustomed to frank discussions with patients regarding their sexual activities. After all, I was a "bone" doctor, not a gynecologist or a urologist!

The other part of the problem was that I did not know that much about back pain and sex. Certainly I knew about back pain, and I had some knowledge about "sexology," but I had not had a great deal of experience in relating one to the other. Over the years, my patients have taken care of both problems. The old adage "When you listen, you learn" certainly applied in this instance. When my back patients would bring up the problem, I would simply say, "Tell me about it." If I made them feel comfortable, they would talk freely, and I would listen. They needed information and understanding, not any judgmental statements or sermons from me.

Although people come in all sizes, shapes, colors, and persuasions, they are basically alike. All people require food, shelter, and clothing. All of us need human contact. We all experience basic human emotions like love and hate, sadness and joy, and serenity and anger. The most elemental of all emotions is the sexual drive or desire, without which the human race would not continue. All animals have a sexual drive, but in humans sex has become more than a procreational activity. It has become intertwined with our personalities, our striving for success, our sense of acceptance, and our need for recognition.

I am not a psychiatrist or a sexual therapist. I am an orthopedic surgeon who takes care of people with back problems and who has developed a great deal of understanding of their back pain and the other anxieties that accompany that complex problem.

So, what about sex and the back? First of all, people with back problems certainly can have satisfactory sexual relations. Obviously if someone is writhing on the floor in agony with back pain or has shooting electrical shocks in the leg, having sex is not uppermost in his or her mind! Furthermore, if you arrive home in the morning after having back surgery, be assured that you will want a little peace and quiet in bed that night. Those are the extreme and usually infrequent times when your back can truly prohibit sexual activities. On the other hand, a bad episode of back pain does not preclude "a little loving." While certain positions of sexual intercourse can exacerbate an existing back problem, or can precipitate a severe spasm in a weak or unstable back, there are also safe and comfortable positions that allow you to fully enjoy the pleasures of making love without the fear of damaging your back. I shall describe a few of these positions for you, but remember this is not a sex manual, and my discussion will relate more to your back movements than to intimate details of making love.

Before continuing, you should be aware that any type of pain can diminish your ardor or cool your sexual passion. It does not have to be back pain. If you realize that, part of your anxieties and fears can be alleviated. It is normal not to become sexually aroused when you are in acute pain. Mother Nature has other things in mind for you. So rest easy, there is nothing wrong with your sex drive that a little relief from back pain will not cure. The "mental" aspects of sex are often much more disabling and more often responsible for loss of libido and impotency than are physical problems. With that understood, I can now proceed with sex and your back.

Gymnastic or acrobatic sexual activities are not appropriate for back-pain sufferers. I have a vivid imagination, but there are some things I have heard and read about that exceed it. Variety in sexual activity is healthy and fun, just as long as it does not hurt or injure either party. So we come to back pain and sex. Rule One is that as long as it does not hurt, it is okay. If you have already found positions that do not cause or aggravate back problems, then you are not in need of the remainder of this discussion. But if you do not fall into that category and are fearful of sexual activities, read on.

The lower back is intimately involved in sexual activity. Pelvic motions occur through the lower back and the hip joints. Men and women alike use this pelvic motion in sexual activity not only to achieve their own sensations, but also to gratify their sexual partners as well. Controlling pelvic movement is a learned skill. Belly dancers were not born with the knowledge or ability to roll and undulate the pelvis. They were taught these motions and practiced them in order to become expert and graceful. Extension and flexion of the lower spine causes the pelvis to move backward or forward. The stomach and buttock muscles control that movement. Side-to-side and rolling motions of the pelvis are accomplished by a combination of the hip and lower-back and stomach muscles.

"Stop here," says the back sufferer. "The idea of trying to move my pelvis around brings tears to my eyes." Well, that may be true, at least partially true. If you have back spasms, the ability to move your pelvis is limited, and many positions of sexual intercourse will be impossible. Since your pelvic mobility is limited, and in the midst of your sexual excitement you do not want to be carried away and do something extreme (as in the example I cited earlier), you want to be in a position that is safe and controlled. This applies equally to men and women.

Usually it is the extension motion of the pelvis that can irritate or stress the lower back; the movement in which the buttocks are brought backward, exaggerating the lumbar lordosis or swayback position of the spine. Forward movement of the pelvis is comfortable and actually eases stress and pain in the lumbar region. Hence, positions that facilitate the forward movement of the pelvis and eliminate or diminish the backward motion are those that you will find most comfortable for your back during sexual activity.

All standing or sitting positions should be automatically eliminated because of the pressure of gravity and lack of support for your back. If you are going to make love, do it lying down, preferably on a firm surface. A soft mattress or couch allows too much of a sag in the lower back, which can cause additional strain and also can diminish the participants' abilities to interact with each other. The floor is always a safe place. As far as the backseat of the car is concerned, I would advise you to put your desire on hold until you can find a more appropriate setting. One of my patients was carried away with passion in the backseat of a car and found herself in a hospital bed the next day. There are times when discretion is the better part of ardor.

The sexual partner with a bad back should assume the bottom position, with his or her partner on top. When lying on your back with the knees bent, your lumbar spine is at rest and is protected. Moving the pelvis forward from this position is not dangerous, and the rhythm of bringing the pelvis forward and allowing it to drop back can be established. Actually this mimics exactly the pelvic-roll exercise that I describe in the section on exercises. With this movement, you are not only enjoying sex, but you are also exercising your back. Since it is so beneficial, maybe you should do it more often!

Meanwhile, the partner on top can be more vigorous but should exert some caution. A large man should remember that a "gentleman rests on his elbow" so that the lady beneath him is not crushed by his weight, especially if she has a bad back. When the man is on the bottom, the female partner has the upper hand and controls the rate and vigor of the activity. The man in this position can rest his back and exercise his pelvic roll.

The face-to-face side position is usually too uncomfortable for the back-pain sufferer. If you both lie with your legs straight, contact and penetration are very difficult. If the woman places her leg underneath her partner's hip, that could aggravate his aching back, and if she tried to move her pelvis in that position, it would send a few alarm signals into her aching back.

The side position in which the woman faces away and the man snuggles against her back is probably the safest, most comfortable, and most satisfying position in which to make love when one or both parties have back problems. The woman flexes her hips and knees and the man snuggles against her, his chest and stomach against her back and his thighs and knees against the back of her thighs and knees. Both partners are thus in a partial fetal position, and as you know by now, the fetal position is the best attitude for your back when lying down. In this position, penetration is easily accomplished, and the forward and backward movement of the pelvis can be maintained without strain.

I am often asked, "When is it safe to resume sexual activities after a bad episode of back or sciatic pain?" The answer is relatively simple—use common sense. If your back is still in spasm and you are taking pain relievers, it's not a good time to make love. A woman cannot relax and participate if her back is in spasm, and a man's ardor will be quickly deflated by an agonizing movement. There is always "later or tomorrow," so be sensible and patient, and when you do feel better, use one of the safe positions that I have described. Eventually, when your back is better, you will be able to resume those positions and activities that you most enjoy.

The same is true after back surgery. Patients are discharged only a few days after having a herniated disk removed. It takes time for healing to occur, and for the first three weeks special precautions are necessary. Once again, if the urge is great and cannot be denied, you can satisfy your desires if you are sensible and careful.

As men reach the end of their fifties, there is a natural lessening of their sexual drives. According to the experts, the sexual drive is strongest in men from eighteen to thirty-five years of age and is most intense in women from thirty to fifty years of age. The reason I mention age and sex drive is that spinal problems can cause difficulty with sexual functions. Although it is very rare, a herniated disk can pinch the nerves that supply the genital area. This can cause numbness in the vaginal area in women and impotency in men. Usually removal of the disk and subsequent relief of pressure on the nerve roots allow normal function to return.

In middle-aged men, spinal stenosis can cause constriction of the same nerves and produce subtle changes. Differentiating problems such as the loss of libido or difficulty in having and sustaining an erection, which accompany changes of life, from a problem of nerve-root compression caused by spinal stenosis can be perplexing. Whenever this problem is brought to my attention, I suggest a urological consultation. Tests are available to determine the cause of the impotency. Actually it is most unusual for impotency to be caused by spinal nerve-root compression. More often it is related to emotional factors and advancing age. Today, there are treatments that can be helpful in both these latter instances. Although earlier I said that impotency was rarely associated with spinal stenosis, I have several male patients who have noted an improvement in their sexual activity after surgical decompression was performed. Whether or not the improvement was due to decompression of the nerve roots themselves, or just the relief from pain and discomfort, I am unable to determine. The bottom line is that their sexual activity improved. In no way would I ever suggest that a decompression laminectomy would improve an individual's sex life. If the operation is needed, it is necessary because of pain and paralysis. If your sexual activities are diminished because of spinal stenosis, improvement in that area is possible with surgery, but never anticipate, never expect that impotency will be improved by having a back operation alone.

NO MORE ACHING BACK

Back pain and sex are closely related subjects, and problems which can easily bring havoc to your self-esteem and relationships. I have tried to be open and candid in my explanations, without being too technical or offensive in any way. A little humor always helps to ease embarrassment when discussing problems that strike close to the heart. I hope this section has helped you. If you do have problems in this area beyond the scope of this book, then I urge you to discuss them frankly with your doctor.

8. Exercise and Sports for Health

Exercise to heal, strengthen, and protect your back is the major emphasis of this book. I know from personal experience and from the experiences of thousands of patients how effective a simple exercise program can be in promoting the health of your back. However, back exercises alone do not give you an overall healthy body or improve your general endurance or stamina. Other types of exercise, such as aerobic exercises to improve your cardiac and pulmonary function, are needed for that purpose. Exercise helps to correct high blood pressure, and it certainly helps in keeping your weight down. By improving your overall body condition, you not only strengthen your heart, but you also increase your body stamina and can work longer without getting tired. Your mind will seem keener, and you will concentrate better. A sense of well-being is another benefit of exercise. Your mood is happier and you are more relaxed and at ease when you exercise regularly.

Whenever I start to get grouchy, my wife sends me out to play squash or tennis. She knows that when I return after playing, I am relaxed and easier to live with. Why does this happen? Why is exercise so good for you? The obvious answer is that when your body is in good condition, you feel healthy and vigorous. Your body works better, and there is a definite spring to your walk. The other, less obvious answer is that exercising and raising your pulse rate above 120 for thirty minutes or more exercises not only your heart, lungs, and muscles but also your metabolic and hormonal systems. Exercise burns off the excess adrenaline in your system that has accumulated as the result of various frustrations during the day. You feel less tense and edgy when your adrenaline levels are lower. Exercise stimulates the production of endorphins, the newly discovered hormones that act upon the brain to decrease pain sensation and to give you a sense of euphoria—a natural high. Runners frequently tell me that after three to four miles they suddenly get a "high" feeling—a sense of euphoria and well-being. This feeling comes from the secretion of endorphins into the bloodstream and can carry over into your daily life.

EXERCISE

If exercise is so good, why doesn't everyone do it? Mostly because it takes time and effort, especially when you first start out. It is hard to do, and your muscles ache after you use them. Your stamina is limited, and you feel tired afterward. The amazing paradox of exercise is that you may begin a session feeling weary and sort of "down," and end up sweating and puffing but happy and relaxed. While exercises are vital for good health, the key is to do them regularly in spite of all conflicts and excuses, and to get on a program that is appropriate for you.

Back-pain sufferers can do general exercises and participate in sports without aggravating or further injuring their lower backs. Before they embark upon any exercise or athletic project, however, their backs must be in good shape. They should have been on a program of back exercises that they can do with ease (I shall describe this program later). When they have accomplished that, they are ready to start on a general exercise program for health and for fun.

General body conditioning involves either an aerobic-exercise program or various sports. Certain of these activities can adversely affect your back. I shall discuss the various exercises that are potentially harmful and potentially good for your back. For the most part, as long as you do the general body exercises properly with some simple modifications, which I shall mention, you will have minimal restrictions.

General Body Exercises

Stretching and aerobic classes are available for all ages in nearly every community, large and small, across the country, from the local community center to the fancy health clubs. These usually consist of general stretching exercises to improve your limberness, and a series of rapid movements or thrusts for strengthening your muscles and raising your heart rate. Often a certain amount of jumping or dancelike movements are incorporated into the program. When attempting these programs or yoga-type exercises, back sufferers should avoid activities that are associated with bending of the spine unless the knees are bent as well. They should also avoid hyperextension exercises in which you arch backward over your pelvis, particularly if that is done with any force. These movements have the potential to aggravate or re-injure an old back problem. Jumping, hopping, or running activities that are considered to be jarring exercises can also exert a considerable impact on your lower back. Should you avoid these exercises entirely? No, but approach them cautiously and caefully. Work your way slowly into a program. If your back starts to ache either during or after the activity, that exercise may not be for you. Do not be discouraged. Although you may not be able to do certain specific exercises or movements, there are many more you can do without hurting your back and still achieve your goal of body limberness and stamina improvement.

Running

Americans have discovered running, and a new industry has been built around it. Marathons have become numerous in the United States and around the world. People everywhere are getting into the act. Years ago, I would prohibit my back patients from running. I was certain that the steady impact of the foot against the ground would send shock waves to the lower back and further injure the already damaged disk or arthritic facet joint. If patients insisted on running, I advised them to run on their toes in order to soften the impact. Well, since then I have learned a great deal about running, especially from my patients. I no longer unconditionally stop patients from running. I have patients upon whom I have operated, both for removal of herniated disks and even for spine fusions, who have since participated in marathons without any back problems. On the other hand, many of my patients experience back or leg pain by simply running for a bus.

The decision to run rests with you. How much does it mean to you, and how dedicated are you to running? If you are determined to run, a few words of advice are in order. You already probably know that you should wear good running shoes, try to run on soft surfaces (not hard pavement) and stretch well before and after you run. Long-distance runners do not run on their toes but rather run with their feet relatively flat. If you are just starting to run, begin gradually and build up the distance slowly. Do not run for speed, but only for distance. Speed running intensifies the impact on your back, and is almost certain to have a deleterious affect. Running every other day, especially in the beginning, gives your body a day to recover before you stress it again. Take the time to learn how to run properly by talking to experts and reading informative books and articles on the subject.

If you have good knees and hips, running is wonderful exercise. You can run almost anywhere in the world, and you do not need special equipment. For some people, running comes easily and naturally, and for others running is more difficult, particularly in the beginning. Nevertheless, everyone can enjoy it and its healthful effects on the body. Thus, if you have the desire to run, try it, but do begin slowly. If pain ensues, then it would be wise to switch to another type of exercise before you cause any significant damage.

Exercise Machines

The emphasis on cardiovascular and pulmonary fitness has led to an explosion of exercise machines: stationary bicycles, treadmills, rowing machines, cross-country ski machines, and the Stairmaster can be seen in health clubs and gymnasiums throughout the world. One or more of these have become permanent fixtures in many homes. Actually they are all good devices to exercise your body in the confines of your home or at the gym. The rate at which you move or work is dependent upon your ability, strength, and endurance. I am in favor of using these machines because they are an efficient way to exercise your body, are not dependent upon the weather, are readily available in your home or gym, and can be adjusted according to individual needs.

Back sufferers, however, must approach these machines with caution. If your back is adversely affected by sitting, an exercise bike might not be suitable for you. Rowing machines produce a great deal of stress on the lower back and on the hamstrings. Generally this machine should be avoided by people with back problems. However, a few of my back patients are rowing enthusiasts, and they work on the machine without pain or spasm. If you plan to use a rowing machine, you must stretch your hamstrings and make certain that they are not tight; otherwise you are sure to injure your back.

Treadmills have the same effect on the lower back as running. There is an impact that flows up to the lower back as the foot strikes the ground, and even fast walking on the treadmill can cause that impact. However, as I mentioned earlier in this section, many of my back patients tolerate both outdoor running and running on a treadmill without ill effects. Once again, if it does not hurt, it is okay to do. Pain is a reliable indicator.

An outgrowth of the treadmill is the Stairmaster. This machine has revolving steps. You keep walking up steps but stay in one place. It is more strenuous than a treadmill, but does not cause impact on your back. I have not tried this machine myself, but theoretically it should not be harmful to your lower back.

The cross-country ski machine is probably the best all-around machine for aerobic exercise and has the least potential for injury to the lower back. The movements of the legs are all gliding and under control. There is no impact involved. The muscles of the buttocks, legs, and stomach are all made to work, and thus are strengthened. Using the hand-pulley ropes provides excellent exercises for the upper body and is of additional benefit to the heart and lungs.

Numerous Nautilus and muscle-building exercise machines are available for working out. For the most part, if reasonable weights and resistance are used, the person with back problems can manage most of these machines. However, before working with any of this equipment, talk to the trainer or therapist in charge of the unit. Inform him or her of your back problems, and let the trainer select which machines you should use and how to use them properly. The improper use of any of this equipment can result in an injury, and if your back is susceptible, it could create a serious problem.

Weight lifting is generally contraindicated for bad backs. Bench presses, lying on your back with your knees bent and lifting weights, are probably the least dangerous for your back, but should be done cautiously and not with excessive weights. For the most part, I advise against weight lifting for my patients.

In recent years, new machines and equipment have been especially developed to strengthen the muscles associated with the spine, particularly those muscles that extend the spine. These machines are also being used to assess the strength of the back muscles. These machines are not for use at home and should be used only under the supervision of a therapist.

Skiing

Surprising as it may seem, skiing is not a bad exercise for the back. Many people are worried that if they take a bad fall, they can injure their backs, but falling while skiing rarely causes back injuries. The actual position in which one skis, with hips and knees flexed and body weight forward, is a safe and protected position for the lower back. The problems come when people start to do "mogul jumps" or fly down hills at excessive speeds. When you are out of control down a steep mountain, it is not your back you have to worry about, it is your life. However, if you are a prudent skier, then I would encourage you to enjoy it without fear or anxiety. Downhill skiing is exhilarating and requires strong legs. It is essential that you exercise and strengthen your legs before you do downhill skiing.

Cross-country skiing is a much more strenuous and beneficial exercise because it requires entire body effort to move along on a level plain, and it is least hazardous to the back. Although you may not have the excitement of speed, you do have the satisfaction of gliding through the snow and utilizing your whole body in this sport.

Horseback Riding

Not long ago, I was examining a twelve-year-old girl who was trying to hide the fact that she had back pain. She was an avid equestrian and had recently taken a fall. Her mother noted she seemed to have trouble straightening up and moving about. When asked if anything hurt, the girl would vehemently deny it, yet at times she appeared to have tears in her eyes. Indeed, when I examined her, I did find that she had tenderness in her spine, and certain motions were obviously painful. I took an X-ray of her back and discovered that she had a small crack in one of her vertebral bones. Upon further questioning, she admitted that she had taken a bad fall from the horse and got back on without telling anyone about it. She was fearful that because of the accident, her parents would forbid her to ride again. Well, I spoke with the child and her parents. I informed them that the fracture was simple and that it would heal. As for returning to horseback riding, I personally saw no reason why she could not.

Except for any injury that can occur when you are thrown from a horse, horseback riding in itself does not cause back problems. A good rider rarely hits the saddle with a significant impact. When someone rides with an English saddle, the rider is posting, and when the horse moves in a rapid trot or gallop, the rider's legs are doing the work. In addition, the upper body is held rigidly erect. Thus, this activity holds the spine in good posture and builds up the muscles that support it. Almost all of my patients who have had lower-back problems and who love horseback riding have been able to return to their favorite pastime. An essential requirement is that they perform their back exercises every day. But that is true for all back sufferers, regardless of the sport or activity in which they like to participate.

Skating

Roller skating and ice skating are two activities which are becoming increasingly popular. The fluid motion of gliding over surfaces can be exhilarating. Most people with back problems safely enjoy skating. Potential injury to the back by falling is relatively rare. However, anyone with brittle or osteoporotic bones should be wary of skating because a hard fall could result in a broken bone. Both ice and roller skating are good forms of general exercise. For the beginners I would advise extra padding on elbows and knees. Because considerable stress is placed upon the hamstrings and heelcords, it is important that sufficient time be given to stretch those particular muscles before the activity is begun.

Dancing

I am often asked about the exercise value of dancing. Although dancing is a relaxing and enjoyable activity, both the old-fashioned ballroom and disco varieties, it is not a very effective exercise for either strengthening the back or improving endurance. Nevertheless, because dancing does involve active body motions and is also great fun, I certainly encourage those of you who like this activity to participate enthusiastically. Disco dancing may involve rather strenuous twisting of the lower back, but if done with the knees bent and in time with the music, it should not excessively strain your lower back.

Ballet, modern dance, and jazz dancing require more intensive stretching of the back and legs. If you are supple, these activities should be easily tolerated. However, if your back is vulnerable, you must be cautious in how vigorously you participate, particularly with the quick shifting movements associated with modern or jazz dancing. Sudden hyperextension or backward arching of the spine is particularly dangerous and should be avoided or at least not carried to an extreme.

Walking

Not everyone enjoys athletics or working out. Furthermore, many of you do not have the time or money to attend special classes or go to a health club or a gym. But everyone can walk, and walking is an excellent aerobic exercise. It can be done almost anywhere, requires no special equipment except comfortable shoes, and the time can be adjusted to fit your busy schedule. Many people tell me that they walk all the time, implying that they are exercising all the time. However, the walking they do most of the day is done in short spurts: across the room, up and down steps, a few blocks to the store, etc. That type of short duration walking is really not exercise. Walking as an exercise requires time and concentration. A leisurely stroll in the park or down a busy thoroughfare, stopping frequently to gaze into store windows requires very little effort. Walking for exercise must be performed at a brisk steady pace for at least thirty minutes. If you are just beginning a walking program, it is wise to start gradually with shorter distances, but as your stamina improves, to maintain a brisk walk for two to three miles or thirty to forty-five minutes. Exercise studies have demonstrated that brisk continuous walking is as beneficial for your heart and lungs as jogging. So for those of you who disclaim any inclination to be athletic, walking is an excellent alternative.

Swimming

I saved swimming for last in this section on exercise. Everyone agrees that swimming is the best and safest aerobic exercise of all. However, that is not necessarily true for all people with back problems. First of all, most people swim on their stomachs and use either a crawl or breaststroke, both of which cause hyperextension of the lumbar spine. After a recent episode of back pain, or after recent surgery, swimming prone or on your stomach should be avoided because of the strain it places on your lower back. Innumerable patients have complained to me about pain when swimming despite having been told by the experts that swimming is the best exercise for the back. These patients developed more pain and discomfort than when they started. It is not that swimming is bad, but that certain positions in swimming are bad.

Here we are talking about posture again. Remember those explanations about back pain being associated with bad posture, whether sitting, standing or lying down? Well those dicta apply even to swimming. If your back is painful or even just aching and stiff, avoid swimming on your stomach. Use a sidestroke or an elementary backstroke, which has a lateral motion (not one in wich you reach back over your head). You can then experience the benefit of exercising in the water without straining your back. Simple logic and good old common sense goes a long way. If you understand your back, you should know what you can and cannot do.

By the way, I am often asked if it is advisable to swim only in warm water. The answer is a simple "no." It is the swimming, and not the temperature of the water, which is important.

Sports and Athletics

Solitary exercise programs are good for the body and for your general health, though for some people they lack the excitement and sociability of sports. Since I encourage my patients to participate in sports, I shall make some general statements about how to reconcile them with your back problems and what precautions you must take.

In general, except for vigorous contact sports such as tackle football or rugby, there is no sport that is totally prohibited to the back patient. Some sports are more likely to cause back problems than others, and if not entirely avoided, participation should at least be carefully limited.

Bowling is a very popular sport. It is one of those activities in which the social aspects are as important as actually throwing the ball down the lane. However, even though the body position of bowling, in which the knees and hips are flexed and the back is bent forward slightly, is generally a good safe position in which the back can function, the unevenness of the throw caused by the heavy weight of the ball in one hand can produce pains in the lower back. If you are not a frequent bowler and have back problems, I would recommend that you avoid this sport. However, if you bowl regularly and have back problems and yet wish to continue, then it is important that you strengthen your back and perhaps alter your swing in order to relieve pressure on your spine.

Basketball is another sport that should be limited. A casual game without too much running is not harmful. An intense game with jumping, extending the spine, landing hard on your heels, and sudden twisting motions can lead to serious injury to the back and disks.

Volleyball is similar to basketball in its effect on the back. A light game without extreme intensity is enjoyable. The point is to keep it competitive but fun. The same applies to soccer and to lacrosse.

Baseball, America's favorite pastime sport, played by young and old alike, is not usually detrimental to the lower back. Because the pace of the game is rather slow, and accompanied by periods of inactivity (except for the pitcher and the catcher), the weekend baseball player does not have to be in great shape. Running is generally done in spurts, and unless you hit a home run, you rarely get out of breath. However, a lusty swing of the bat is associated with considerable twisting of the lower spine, and your lower back is especially vulnerable to twisting motions. If you are sensible about the degree of intensity with which you compete and keep your back in good shape, you should be able to play baseball, particularly softball, safely and without concern.

Racquet sports have gained enormous popularity. People are playing squash, tennis, racquetball, and paddle tennis in greater numbers than ever before. Ping-Pong and badminton are less strenuous. Racquet sports are similar in the stresses they place on the body and the lower back, except for Ping-Pong, which is almost entirely a wrist game. But you should be aware that Ping-Pong also has twisting, lunging movements involving the back.

Surprisingly, racquet sports are not usually strenuous on the lower back. The proper body stance when playing is with your knees slightly bent and your body weight forward. This position protects your lower back, encouraging the use of your legs and hips. There are two movements that are potentially dangerous in tennis. One is the overhead smash in which the lower back arches backward as the racquet is brought to full height. Hyperextension is always dangerous for the lower back. Be careful when hitting that overhead shot not to arch your back excessively. The same is true of the serve. Throw the ball over your front foot, and that decreases the degree of backward extension of your spine.

The other movement that could cause problems with your back is the twisting motion of the trunk, usually associated with an awkward backhand swing. If you remember to keep your knees bent and your body weight evenly distributed, you can avoid hurting your back.

Because of my own back problems, for many years I avoided tennis and squash. However, with just those few adjustments, I am able to play to my heart's content, or at least to my present level of endurance. I do my back exercises every day, and I am able to play with confidence that I will not be hurting my back. Daily exercises are essential, as I learned the hard and painful way. I admit shamefully that at times in the past, because of various time restrictions, I did not exercise as regularly as I should have. Whenever I did not exercise every day, I began to feel some soreness, stiffness, or pain in my back, which was exacerbated when I played squash or tennis. I paid the penalty with not only pain in my back (in my case, sciatic pain as well) but also time lost from work while I was recuperating in bed. I know that it is only human to avoid doing routine exercises in the morning when you feel well, but after you have experienced the painful lesson a few times, boring or not, you learn to do the exercises. I hope that you, my readers, will heed this advice and will not have to learn the lesson the hard way.

Another thing to avoid is playing tennis on a hard surface. A hard surface, even a rubberized one, is strenuous not only on your back but also on your hips and knees. Countless patients have arrived in my office after a wonderful weekend of tennis, complaining of aching backs and knees. Questioning reveals that they were playing on hard surfaces. The problem with the hard surface is not that it is hard, but that you cannot slide. As you run to the ball and plant your foot, soft surfaces, such as grass, clay, Astroturf, or artificial turf, allow the foot to slide an inch or two, which eases the impact on your knees and back. On a hard-surface court, when you plant that foot, it stops there, and the impact travels to your knees, hips and back. Younger people have no problem with hard surfaces, but after age fifty those hard surfaces take their toll. My advice is to play on soft surfaces whenever possible, or if playing on a hard surface, it would be better to play every other day, thereby resting your back between sessions.

Golf is another game that requires a good deal of twisting of the back. The club swing starts on one shoulder and extends across the body to the back of the other shoulder. When done smoothly, it is a beautiful motion to behold. But there are many a slip and hitch from beginning to end, and a little mishap can trigger an explosion of pain in the lower back. If you are diligent with your back exercises, you are less likely to strain your back while playing golf. A common mistake that golfers (good ones and bad ones) often make occurs after a long absence from the game such as over the winter months, or after an illness or a prolonged back attack. Because they have not played in a long time, they are eager to get their swing back in the groove. Off they go to a golf range and hit basket after basket of balls, trying every club in their bag. This excessive swinging, using muscles and joints, especially in the back and shoulders, that are a bit rusty, can inflame even a healthy back, and can be devastating to a vulnerable back.

Golf is a wonderful sport, and if you love it, I would encourage you to play. Be sensible, though. Do your back exercises and try to play with a relaxed attitude. You are most likely to hurt your back with long drives, especially if you are trying for extra yards. That extra effort in your swing might be too much for your back. A bit of sage advice that I give to my patients is to try to hit the ball twenty yards less than normal, regardless of what club they use (except for the putter, of course). If they concentrate on hitting the ball squarely, their swing will be smoother, and often the ball goes even farther! Even if the distance is not as great, at least you are able to play golf without back pain.

Additional Advice About Sports and Your Back

After reading this section, you must realize that you can probably participate in any sport you enjoy. You must keep two things in mind if you want to be able to play without back pain. The first is that you must do your back exercises every day on a regular basis; that is a given—an absolute. The second is to put sports in a proper perspective; winning is not everything and not even the only thing, regardless of what Vince Lombardi said. Especially for those of you who have had back problems.

I have to confess that I used to play tennis and squash to win every point. I would often self-destruct with some of the maneuvers I put my body through in order to return the ball or hit a winner. Needless to say, I often paid the price with pain. However, I accepted that as part of the game. I played football in high school and college, and my coaches always preached that you not only played with pain but that it was good for you; it strengthened your character and made a man out of you! Of course, I accepted that as gospel, which was fine when my body was limber, my joints younger, my reactions faster, and my muscles stronger.

Now, pain has a different meaning for me. It informs me that I am overdoing the activity and causing harm to myself. I now heed those warnings. I still may experience some discomfort after a hard match, but that is acceptable. My brother gave me a very important lesson while playing tennis. He taught me to say to my opponent "good shot," instead of trying to chase down and return every single ball. I have learned the lesson, and I still love to play. There comes a time when the important thing is to be able to play, and winning is only secondary. Keep that in mind for the health of your back and your body.

A well-balanced exercise program should involve your daily back exercises, some type of aerobic activity twice weekly, and some type of sport activity twice weekly. Cardiologists state that exercising to raise your heart rate to 120 beats a minute and maintain it for thirty minutes three times a week is very good for your heart and general circulation. At this point, I would like to emphasize very strongly that *if you have a heart condition or any other medical problem, you should consult your doctor before embarking on any exercise program.*

9. First Aid for Your Back

When that first episode of back pain strikes, it can occur at the most unlikely and untimely moment. You may be out of town, it may occur on the weekend or in the evening, or your doctor may be away. If the pain is not severe, you can manage to walk and get from place to place with bearable discomfort, and thus you can wait a day or so before seeing if it is necessary to go to the doctor. But when the pain is disabling or agonizing, you need some guidelines on how to help yourself until you get medical attention.

I am not proposing to make you a back specialist, nor do I think it is wise to treat yourself without expert advice. I do believe, however, that several simple instructions can be of help to you or someone you know who needs relief from back pain.

Back attacks come in all degrees of severity. The milder scenario is pain and stiffness that is localized to the back. This pain may be intermittent and only present when you change positions such as getting up from a chair or bending over to put on your shoes. You may still be able to continue with your normal activities. If the symptoms resolve spontaneously, consider yourself fortunate and begin your back exercises so that the next episode can either be lessened or prevented.

In other instances, the back pain might be considerably more severe and constant. Movements may be very painful and restricted. If the onset of pain is acute, such as that which results from a sneeze or a sudden twist of the back, a cold application to your back can help to decrease the spasms. Lying in bed, either in the fetal position or on your back with your knees elevated by pillows or a bolster, usually eases the pain. Aspirin or anti-inflammatory medication (ibuprofen compounds, of which many are available over the counter) can help to reduce the pain. When the pain is this bad, you should see your doctor as soon as possible. With rest and medication, the attack will subside, and then you can begin the exercise program.

An attack of back pain may be accompanied by a radiation of the pain into your leg. If the pain goes into the thigh but not below the knee, it may *not* be caused by a herniated disk. If the pain goes all the way down the leg to the ankle and foot (classical sciatica) it *is* most likely due to a herniated disk. Get to bed immediately, in either the fetal position or on your back with knees bent. Call your doctor right away. Symptoms may subside in a few days, but if they persist, you will need careful observation and treatment.

I will now summarize the steps you can take to relieve the pain and discomfort of a back problem when a doctor is unavailable. I shall provide guidance for three degrees of pain and discomfort—mild, moderate, and severe.

Mild Pain: Diffuse Aches and Stiffness
1. Do easy limbering and stretching exercises, followed by the regular exercises if the latter are not painful.
2. Take a hot shower.

3. Take aspirin or other anti-inflammatory medications; follow dosage recommended on label.
4. Avoid long car rides or traveling.
5. Be careful when bending and lifting.
6. Don't sit on soft chairs.
7. If your mattress is soft, place a bed board underneath it.
8. Lie on your side in the fetal position or on your back with pillows under your knees.
9. When your back feels tired or aching, lie on the floor with your knees bent.
10. Do a pelvic tilt when standing to ease discomfort and fatigue in the lower back.
11. If the symptoms persist more than a few days, call your doctor.

Moderate Pain: Difficulty in standing straight, pains with movement, able to walk but with discomfort.
1. Give yourself bed rest with pillows under the knees or lying on your side in the fetal position. Put no more than one pillow under your head.
2. Confer with your doctor on the phone.
3. Take aspirin or other anti-inflammatory medications: Follow dosage recommended on the label or by your doctor.
4. Apply ice packs on the lower back (not against bare skin), twenty minutes on, twenty minutes off, for two hours, twice a day.
5. You may get out of bed for bathroom needs, but limit the number of times (maximum four to five times in twenty-four hours).
6. Avoid sitting.
7. Stand for meals—not more than fifteen minutes.
8. Stay home for two days—don't travel unless absolutely necessary.

9. Do no exercises until pain and stiffness have subsided, then gently try a few of the basic back exercises. When these are comfortable to do, then slowly add the next group of exercises.
10. Confer again with your doctor for further instructions.
11. When all pain and stiffness has disappeared, slowly resume your normal exercises and activities.

Severe Pain: Unable to stand because of pain, may have severe leg pain with or without back pain. Coughing and sneezing hurt the back and leg.

1. Give yourself bed rest, pillows under your knees or lying on your side in the fetal position. Put only one pillow under your head.
2. Apply ice packs, (not against bare skin) three times a day, twenty minutes on, twenty minutes off, for two hours.
3. Call your doctor.
4. Take aspirin, anti-inflammatory medications, or other medications your doctor might order.
5. Don't get out of bed, use a urinal—use bathroom only when essential. If pain is too severe to walk, crawl on the floor.
6. If you have to get out of bed, roll to your side and push yourself up sideways. Sit on edge of bed, then stand. Have someone help you stand up.
7. Eat lying down on your side, drink with a straw. Have someone cut your food.
8. Confer again with your doctor. If you have numbness and are unable to move your toes or foot, that is an emergency, and you should be seen as soon as possible. If riding in a car is too painful to contemplate, call an ambulance.
9. If pain subsides after forty-eight hours, try standing and walking for five minutes. If your pain

does not increase, then repeat five minutes of standing and walking later in the day.

10. Gradually increase the time you spend out of bed each day, depending upon your pain. If it reaches the moderate level, you can follow the guidelines for that section. Use common sense with your activities.

11. Confer with your doctor again, either by phone or in his office. He will advise you how to further proceed with your activities.

If you are unable to tolerate aspirin or anti-inflammatory medications because of stomach problems, try Tylenol or a similar compound. Do not take someone else's medication unless you have your doctor's approval. Your neighbor's pain pills or tranquilizers may be safe for him or her but not for you. When in doubt as to what to take, always call your doctor. By the way, you do not have to call the specialist right away. Your own family doctor or internist can analyze your symptoms over the phone and prescribe medication. He knows which medication is safe for you, and he also knows when it is necessary to consult a specialist.

10. My Complete Low-Back Exercise Program

The time has come to describe my exercise program for your back. I have mentioned it all through this book. I have told you why exercises are essential for a healthy back and why they are so important. Now, I shall tell you how to do them properly, how many times to do each exercise, and in what order they should be done. Obviously there are some individuals who cannot do certain exercises. As I describe the exercises, I shall also stress the ones that may be difficult for some of you.

Although almost all back sufferers can do these exercises safely, there will be some for whom the back exercises are not appropriate. Therefore, if you are having or have had special problems with your back or any other medical problems, you must consult your doctor before beginning the exercise program. Explain the program to your doctor or even take the book to him or her so your doctor can actually see the program. You may be allowed to do the entire program, or modifications of certain exercises. Although these exercises have been used successfully for thousands of back sufferers, and to my knowledge have not been harmful if done properly, be safe and check with your doctor first.

This program consists of exercises that are prescribed by many doctors and therapists throughout the world for back problems. I claim no originality. Because of my personal interest, during my many years in the practice of orthopedic surgery I developed my own concepts of the causes and treatments of back problems. Over time I have refined these concepts and the exercises that I believe are essential for a healthy back. What I have done is to evaluate hundreds of different exercises for the back, stomach, and legs, and to decide which ones seem to be the most beneficial. I have listened to the experiences of my patients with their various exercises. Furthermore, I have done all of them myself—that is, tried them out to determine which helped and which could cause trouble. I did them in various positions—lying down, sitting, and standing.

One of the first lessons I learned is that if you give patients too many exercises to do, they will never get them done. Thus, an early principle of mine was to limit the number of required exercises for the patient. That meant getting the most out of the exercises that they did do. The exercises were designed to stretch out tight muscles and ligaments that could exert a harmful effect upon the back, such as excessive lordosis and tight hamstrings, and then strengthen the apdominal, spinal, and buttock muscles that support the spine and pelvis.

Finally, the exercises had to be appropriate for young, healthy athletes and equally appropriate for older people with bad spinal problems. I have weighed all these factors in creating this exercise program, and I have been pleased by the excellent benefits many back sufferers have obtained. What great gratification for me, when a patient tells me that he or she has "no more aching back."

The most difficult problem I face with my patients is not in motivating them to begin the exercises, but to continue with them after they feel better. At first they are eager to begin the program. They want to get better and they want to return to their normal activities, so they are willing to do almost anything, and exercise appears to be an easy solution to their back dilemma.

The exercises are easy, and their backs do get better, but doing a set program of back exercises every day becomes monotonous and boring, expecially if you are feeling well. More often than I like to recall, I have patients start off diligently with their exercises, rid themselves of back pain, resume normal activities, and then become lazy and forget to do their daily regime. They miss a day now and then without any obvious consequences. Pretty soon, they stop the exercises entirely.

A month may go by, even several months, without a twinge of pain. Then, one morning they bend down, and straighten up with pain; or as they tee off on the third hole, they collapse with sudden back spasms; or after driving four hours to visit grandparents, they cannot get out of the car without help. All of these scenarios are much too familiar to me, and my frustration lies in the fact that they are all avoidable. I tell my patients that 90 percent of back problems get well with an exercise program if done regularly. I try a little scare tactic. I take a scalpel from a drawer and show it to the patient. I tell the patient that if she or he does the exercises faithfully, an operation will never be required. On the other hand, I remind the patient, I am an orthopedic surgeon (I stress the word *surgeon*), and operating on backs is one of my special skills. But, I tell the patient, I would much rather avoid the need for my surgical skills and simply treat the painful back with the exercise regime.

"You can lead a horse to water, but you cannot make him drink." Many times have we heard that cliché, but it certainly applies to the person with a back problem. Be smart for yourself; not only do the exercises, but do them every day.

WHEN TO DO YOUR BACK EXERCISES

Generally the exercises should not be done when you are in acute pain. Wait until the pain and spasms have subsided before you begin. By that, I mean wait until you are pain-free for a few days. If you have had sciatic or leg pain, consult your doctor before beginning your exercises. If you have had an injury to your spine, you should have your back examined first before exercising. If you are pregnant or have any medical problems, discuss the exercises with your doctor before you start.

You might ask me if it sensible for you to exercise your back even though you have never had any back problems. My answer of course is, *Yes!* An ounce of prevention is worth a pound of cure. The frequent occurrence of back problems in so many millions of people indicates that it makes very good sense to keep your healthy back healthy at all times. By all means, do the exercises, and protect your back now and in the future.

Being a parent has its moments of despair and triumph. I have been lecturing and writing about back problems since my children were babies. My son was one year old when I was hospitalized with my own herniated disk. Fortunately I recovered without surgery, and I do my exercises every day to keep my back healthy, so he has no recollection of how serious a problem it originally was for me. I knew that as he was growing up, the worse thing I could do was lecture him about his back. After all, I was his dad, not his doctor. However, I hoped that watching me do my exercises every morning, combined with his own good sense, would eventually prompt him to begin the exercise program without my urging or nagging.

We never discussed this issue, but recently my son, who is now a young man, and I had the opportunity to be together on a fishing trip. We shared a cabin, and I was both surprised and delighted that when I got on the floor in the morning to do my back exercises, he was right there beside me. Furthermore, he was not doing them for my benefit, but for the protection of his own back. I was enormously pleased, not so much for my own self-satisfaction, but because I knew that as long as he continued with those exercises, he would never experience the pain and back problems that had once plagued his father.

Included in the "when to do the exercises" lesson is the time of day you should do them. When you first start these exercises, you should do them twice a day, preferably the first thing in the morning and just before you go to bed at night. The purpose of the twice-a-day program is to hasten the improvement in your back: to get those tight ligaments and muscles stretched out faster, and to make those supporting muscles stronger more rapidly. I do not wish to imply that *speed* in performing the exercise program is of the essence. In fact, just the opposite. It is essential to do the exercises slowly and correctly. But if you do the exercises slowly twice a day, you are bound to get better that much faster than if you only did them once a day. After you have been on the twice-a-day program for about three months, you should have achieved the desired stretching and improved muscle strength. From then on, you can do your exercises only once a day. In other words, you have achieved your goals with the twice-daily program; now, you have to maintain what you have gained with a daily program.

The truth is that your back is only as strong as those muscles that support it. Muscle strength is achieved and maintained by exercise. If you stop exercising those muscles, they get weaker. All the other sports and exercises you do may be of great benefit for your general body health, but unless you do exercises specifically for your lower back, those important supporting muscles may get weaker. This is especially true if you have had a back problem in the past. You now understand why I insist upon daily exercises.

When you are on the once-a-day program, I recommend that you do the back exercises first thing in the morning: out of bed, onto the floor, exercise, and then proceed with your day's activities. Although I know that some people function better in the morning and others at night, experience has taught me that unless you exercise first thing in the morning, you are unlikely to exercise at all. Life is busy and hectic. Children's problems come before your own; the work at the office can keep you late at night; after an evening out with friends, the last thing you want to do is lie on the floor and exercise your back when you can barely brush your teeth before dropping into bed. However, if you do your exercises first thing in the morning, they are done and you don't have to worry about them for the rest of the day. Think of your back exercises as an important responsibility; if you don't do them, you are certainly going to have problems with your back that could make you miss work, stay home from school, fail to do your part in the car pool, or even deprive your spouse of conjugal rights. That's right, you have no one to blame except yourself if you have problems with your back. So get on that floor and exercise!

I fully understand the pressures upon your time, which is exactly why I strongly advise that you do the exercises first thing in the morning and get them over and done with. Actually, once you are in the habit of the morning program, you will begin to enjoy the extra sense of suppleness and strength with which you begin your day.

HOW TO DO THE EXERCISES

The first principle is that the exercises should be done slowly and thoroughly. Do not rush through them. I know that there is a tendency to finish them quickly. Resist that temptation. The more thoroughly you do the exercises, the greater the benefit for your back. Once you are familiar with your exercises and are doing all of them, the entire program will take about fifteen minutes. If it takes less than that, you are doing them too fast. However, I do not want you to concentrate on the time it takes to do the exercises, but rather on the right way to do each exercise.

The second principle is that the exercises are all done on the floor, preferably on a carpet or exercise mat. Hard bare floors can be rough on your back. A little cushioning provided by a carpet or mat makes doing the exercises more comfortable. Exercising on a bed or couch is very inefficient. The softness and give of either surface will not provide the firmness and support you need to obtain the maximum benefit from your efforts.

The third principle is to relax when you are exercising. Try to keep your mind calm and your body loose. Lie on the floor in a comfortable position. Most people feel comfortable lying on their backs with their arms at their sides and their knees bent. Older people or individuals with spinal deformities may be more comfortable with a small pillow under their heads. Listenig to the morning news on the radio or some calming music is also conducive to relaxation.

A BRIEF DESCRIPTION OF THE EXERCISES

The exercises are divided into groups: The first is a beginning group that combines stretching and strengthening of your back. This set of exercises is particularly designed for someone recovering from back pain or recovering from surgery. I advise people with special problems to only do the first set of exercises (Group A). Group B exercises are more strenuous but should be suitable for most back patients. These are to be done after Group A exercises have become relatively easy to perform. Finally Group C is an advanced program that may not be appropriate for everyone. These exercises are more strenuous and might be too difficult for some people. When I describe this group of exercises, I shall also discuss the indications and limitations of each.

When starting Group A exercises, do each exercise a few times to familiarize yourself with the actual movements involved. Then go through the first five exercises in Group A, doing each one five times. When you can do each one five times without strain or pain, gradually begin to increase the number of repetitions to ten. When you are able to do all the Group A exercises ten times with ease, then you can begin the exercises in Group B. Add each exercise in Group B one at a time. In other words, start with the first exercise in Group B, perform it five times, and slowly, increase the number of repetitions to ten. When you are able to do the ten repetitions with ease, add the next exercise; begin with five repetitions and again increase to ten. Gradually you will have added all the exercises in Group B. After two or three weeks, you should be able to perform all the exercises in Group A and Group B ten times. Remember, initially the exercises are done twice a day. After you have done the entire program twice daily for three months, you can then continue on a maintenance program once daily.

The Group C exercises are advanced. Some of them may be substituted for exercises in Group A or Group B, or they may be simply added to the program to further strengthen your back and stomach. Because they are more strenuous and they may be too difficult for some of you, I suggest great caution in doing them. People with osteoporosis, prior back surgery, or generalized arthritis should not attempt the exercises in Group C. These advanced exercises are for those younger or middle-aged individuals whose backs can not only take the strain, but who want and need extra strengthening.

THE BACK-EXERCISE PROGRAM

Good morning! At least let us pretend it is morning, and you have had a refreshing night's sleep. You feel eager (did I say eager?) to begin your back-exercise program. The thought, the dream, of being free from back pain is incredibly enticing.

Lie with your back on the floor (remember, on a carpeted floor or an exercise mat). Bend your knees at about a 45-degree angle so that your feet are flat and

RESTING POSITION #19

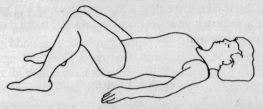

allow your arms to rest comfortably at your sides. (See Figure 19.) If you are uncomfortable lying with your head flat on the floor, use a small pillow under your head. Older people with breathing problems may require a larger pillow.

It is important to "loosen up" before you begin.

- Take a few deep breaths—inhaling and exhaling to a maximum degree.
- Loosen up your neck by rolling it from side to side. When you do this, keep your chin tucked in, move your head slowly, and try to look over the shoulder to which your head is turning. A few turns to each side are all that is necessary.
- Stretch your shoulders by turning your palms and arms in as far as they can go and then reverse the motion, turning the palms and arms out to their maximum excursion. You may feel little popping or cracking noises in your shoulders, but do not worry, you are not injuring yourself. Actually you will find this a very pleasant maneuver.
- Finally reach both arms above your head and, if possible, lay them along the side of your head. In this position, extend your fingers, reach as far behind as you can with one hand, relax that hand and arm, and then repeat on the other side.

175

These first few relaxing and limbering maneuvers should not take more than a few minutes and will help relax and loosen your neck and shoulders for the back-exercise program.

Group A Exercises

Group A consists of five exercises. If you are recovering from a back attack or recuperating from surgery, you have to be especially careful to do each exercise slowly.

If any exercise is painful, and by that I mean something more than stiffness or mild soreness, then stop that exercise. Do the ones that are comfortable for you. After a few days, you may again try the one that initially hurt, and perhaps by that time you can do it without pain. Those of you who are not recovering from a back-pain episode, or who never had a bad aching back, can probably breeze through these first five exercises with ease.

Exercise I: Lower-Back Stretch
(SEE FIGURE 20)

This exercise is designed to stretch your lower back and to improve the mobility of your hips. Bringing your knees to your chest reverses the lordosis of the lumbar spine and stretches those ligaments that tend to cause an exaggeration of that posture. The exercise is done in three parts:

1. Clasp your bent right knee with both hands. Keep your left foot flat on the floor. Bring your right knee toward your chest, but at an angle so that it actually points toward your shoulder. Gently pull the knee back as far as it can go

EXERCISE I #20

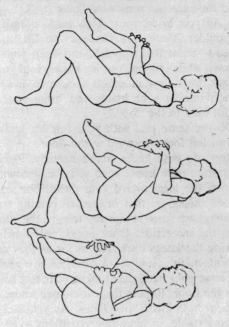

comfortably without pain. If you can reach your shoulder or chest, that is good, but if the structures in your lower back are too tight, you may only be able to bring your knee back partway. Do not be discouraged, because that is normal for many people when they first start this exercise. Gradually over a period of time, your thigh will finally touch your chest. Pulling too hard can stretch the muscles too fast and cause you needless pain and muscle spasm. The key is to pull the thigh to your chest very slowly. Eventually the knee will come back easily, and you can do the exercises somewhat faster.

As you bring your thigh back toward your shoulder, there is a tendency to lift up your head—resist that impulse, and keep your head down while pulling your leg back. Hold your leg back for a few moments (count to five), and then release your hands and bring your right foot back to the floor.

2. Do the same pull with your left leg and bring your left foot backward to the floor.
3. Now, do both knees simultaneously. Place one hand on each knee, keep your head down, and bring the legs toward your chest, but separate your thighs, so that instead of coming straight back, each knee is directed toward the shoulder on the same side. Once again, pull slowly and bring the knees back only as far as they can go comfortably. Hold for a count of five and then release your hands, and allow your feet to come to the floor. Repeat this cycle—one knee, other knee, both knees, five times. As you feel more comfortable, increase the repetitions to ten.

For those of you who have knee problems and who have pain if you pull your knee in the manner described above, there is an important variation that will relieve that strain on the knee. Instead of putting your hands on top of your knee when you pull your leg back, put your hands behind your thigh and allow your knee to bend over your hand. In this position, you can still pull your thigh back, flex your hip, stretch your back, and yet not strain your knee.

Exercise II: Pelvic Roll or Tuck
(SEE FIGURE 21)

Begin with the same position in which you started this exercise program, with your knees bent at a 45-degree angle and arms at the side. Contract your buttocks or gluteal muscles, and slowly lift the edge of your buttocks off the floor. This exercise strengthens your buttock muscles and at the same stretches your lumbar spine. Initially it may feel awkward, as though you have no control of the area. If so, put your legs straight out on the floor and then clench your buttock muscles tightly together. You will find that easy to do. Bend your knees slightly and repeat the tightening of the muscles with your knees slightly bent. Finally return your knees to the original bent position, and by now you should find it easy to perform the buttock tightening.

The pelvic roll or tuck is performed in two steps.

Exercise II #21

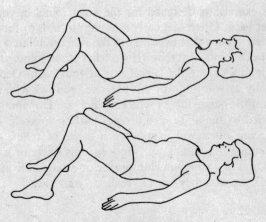

1. The buttock muscles are tightened so that the edge of your buttock rises slowly, yet the lumbar spine stays flat on the floor. Contract your buttocks slowly, and make the actual rise of the pelvis very gradual.
2. Once you achieve maximal contraction of the muscle, hold the tension for a count of five, then slowly allow the muscles to relax and your pelvis to settle against the floor.

This exercise has two major benefits: First, it strengthens the buttock muscles that control your lumbar lordosis, and also you learn how to prevent excessive lordosis when standing, by tightening these same muscles. As noted earlier, doing a pelvic roll or tuck when standing can ease low-back fatigue.

Repeat the exercises five times initially, and then gradually increase to ten times.

Exercise III: Lumbar Spine Twist
(SEE FIGURE 22)

This exercise is designed for the facet joints in your lower back. Often that early morning stiffness or those sudden spasms that twist you to the side are related to the facet joints. Exercise III stretches these joints and the muscles along the lateral side of your back. Occasionally as you perform this exercise, you will experience little snapping or cracking noises. Do not be worried by the noise, you are not hurting yourself. In fact, you often will experience a sense of relief, of something "loosening up." Indeed, this exercise is a variation of a common chiropractic or osteopathic manipulation that they use to "realign" your back.

This exercise must be done cautiously. If you attempt to force the stretch, you may produce the same spasm you are trying to avoid. Follow the instructions carefully.

1. Lie on your back with your knees bent and feet flat on the floor. Place your hands underneath your head, with your fingers intertwined. Bring your shoulder blades together so that your elbows are touching the floor.
2. Cross your bent right leg over your bent left leg and allow both legs to drop toward the right. At the same time, concentrate on keeping your left elbow on the floor. You will experience a stretching sensation along the left side of your body. If you are limber, your legs will touch the floor. Do not force the legs down; allow the weight of your right leg to do the work. Gradually, over time, as you keep stretching, your legs will touch the floor, but even if you are never able to reach the floor with your legs, the exercise is still very beneficial. Remember, do not force the leg downward.

   When your legs have dropped to the side as far as they can, hold that position for a count of five, then bring your legs to the starting cross position and repeat the exercise five times on the right side.
3. Recross your legs, left leg over the right, and do the same exercise on the left side five times.

When you are able to do this exercise comfortably five times on each side, increase the repetitions to ten times each side.

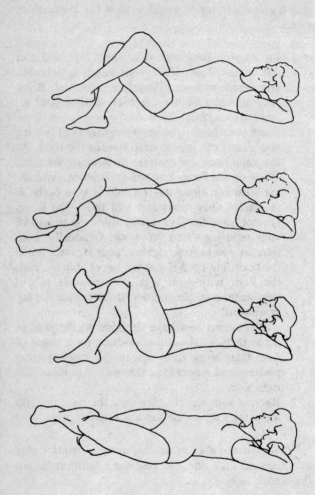

Exercise IV: Single-Leg Lift
(SEE FIGURE 23)

As I have emphasized earlier in this book, tight hamstrings are often the culprit in causing low-back problems. It is essential that the hamstrings are properly stretched. The wrong way to stretch your hamstrings is to stand up and bend over with your knees straight, trying to touch your toes. If your hamstrings are tight and you have had an aching back, this exercise is certain to cause you trouble. Sitting on the floor with yor legs stretched out in front of you, and then bending forward, again trying to touch your toes, is equally bad. In both instances, you are using your back as a lever to stretch your hamstrings, placing an enormous stress on your vulnerable area. I strongly advise you against stretching your hamstrings with either of those exercises.

The safe way to stretch your hamstrings is with your back at rest on the floor, and that is the basis for Exercise IV, the straight-leg lift.

1. Lie on your back with your knees bent, and hands resting at your side. Straighten your right knee, but keep your left knee bent. Stiffen your right thigh muscles so that your right knee is held rigid. Point your toes toward the ceiling. Keeping your right knee stiff and your left knee bent, slowly raise your right leg off the floor. Lift it as high as you can without pain. If your hamstrings are loose, you can bring your leg to a 90-degree angle with your body. If your hamstrings are tight, you may only be able to lift it halfway up. No need for despair if you cannot reach the 90-degree angle immediately—after all, Rome was not built in one day—and if you keep

EXERCISE IV #23

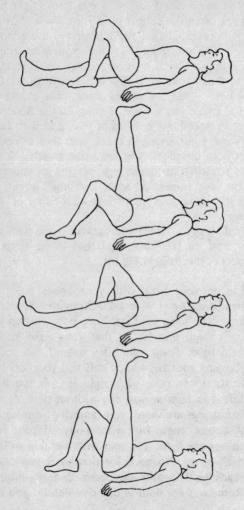

exercising, eventually your hamstrings will stretch, and you will lift your leg easily. If you attempt to stretch the tight hamstrings too strenuously or too rapidly, you can only cause harm and pain.

2. Once you have lifted your leg to the maximum comfortable height, hold it for a count of five, then allow the leg to slowly descend to the floor. Remember to hold your knee quite straight, without bending, in order to achieve the maximum stretching effect upon your hamstrings. If you allow the knee to bend as you lift the leg, you are not accomplishing any further stretching. Keep the knee straight.

An additional advantage of keeping the knee straight is that the sustained contraction of the thigh muscles (the quadricep muscles) builds their strength. Not only do you stretch your hamstrings, but you strengthen your quadriceps at the same time. This will be a help for those of you who are bike riders or skiers.

After you have completed five leg lifts on the right leg, perform the exercise on the left leg. While you are exercising the left leg and hamstrings, remember to keep the right knee bent annd right foot flat.

One last point before proceeding to the next exercise. At the beginning of the exercise, I stress keeping your toes up and back. Holding this position as you lift your leg helps not only your hamstrings but also stretches your heel cords. This exercise may initially appear quite simple, but if it is done properly you achieve three goals: hamstring stretching, quadriceps strengthening, and heel-cord stretching.

When you are able to do five leg lifts on each side without discomfort, regardless of how high you lift the leg, gradually increase the repetitions to ten on each side.

Exercise V: Modified Sit-Up
(SEE FIGURE 24)

The best way to strengthen your stomach muscles is by sit-ups. At gym classes in school, someone would hold your feet, and with your hands behind your head you would raise your body repeatedly until your stomach muscles hurt. That does build stomach muscles, but people with back problems have learned, the hard and painful way, that the old standard sit-up is murder for their backs. What a dilemma! Strong stomach muscles are critical for a healthy back, yet sit-ups aggravate back problems.

The solution to this problem is to do sit-ups with your knees bent. As soon as you modify the exercise this way, you remove the stress on your back, and you can strengthen your stomach muscles without the risk of straining your back.

Research into strengthening stomach muscles has demonstrated that it is not necessary for the body to come all the way up in order for these muscles to work their hardest. If you bring the upper body halfway, the tension and strengthening effect are enough. At the same time, keeping your lower back on the floor prevents straining in that area.

In the beginning of this program, I want you to do the sit-up exercise exactly as I describe it here. Later, if you desire and are able to strengthen those muscles even more, you can add the stomach exercises I describe in Group C.

1. Lie on the floor with your knees bent and your hands resting on your chest. Do a pelvic roll as described in Exercise II, and hold the position.
2. Lift your head and shoulders off the floor, and slowly slide your hands to the top of your knees.

EXERCISE V #24

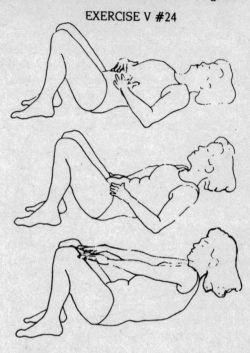

Hold this position for a count of five, then slowly slide your hands back to your chest.

3. Allow your head and shoulders to lie back on the floor, and relax your pelvis. Begin this exercise with five repetitions, and increase to a minimum of ten repetitions.

Some of my patients (including me) do as many as fifty of these modified sit-ups. It is a very effective exercise, and remember, you do not have to bring your chest all the way to your knees—halfway is just as effective.

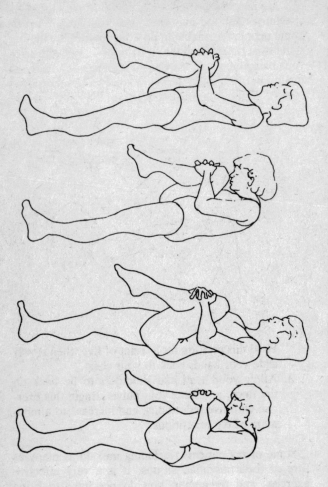

That concludes Group A exercises, the beginning exercise program. After you are able to do each exercise ten times, you may then proceed with Group B. Some people are unable to do Exercise III, the lumbar spine twist. If you find that it irritates or causes pain in your back, eliminate it from the exercise program and just do exercise I, II, IV, V. When you have achieved ease in performing this latter group, then you can still proceed to the exercises in Group B.

Group B: Intermediate Exercises

These four exercises are more strenuous than Group A, but they also further strengthen your muscles. Some of you may not tolerate this group of exercises, because your backs and joints are just too vulnerable. Working with Group A exercises is beneficial, but the increased strain with the Group B exercises may cause pain and discomfort. If that is your situation, remember that half a loaf is better than none. You will still be helped by the exercises in Group A. In fact, you may want to increase the repetitions of each exercise, which is certainly fine if your time permits. Please note that the increased number of repetitions do not replace the benefit of a daily routine. Doubling the exercises three times a week is not as good for you as the usual repetitions seven days a week.

Exercise VI: The First Exercise in Group B
(SEE FIGURE 25)

This exercise will strengthen your stomach muscles and improve the mobility of your hips and upper back and neck.

1. Lie on your back in the usual position. Extend or straighten your left knee until the leg is flat

on the floor. Bring your right knee to your chest with both hands. Keep your head down.

2. Concentrate on keeping your left leg flat on the floor in the straight position, and holding your right thigh against your chest. Bring your head up until you can touch your nose to your knee. Count to five and slowly let your head down. Keep your thigh against your chest and repeat the procedure five times on your right leg.

3. Reverse legs, the right down, the left leg held against your chest, and repeat the same nose-to-knee maneuver five times.

This exercise requires considerable mobility in the upper back and neck. If you are unable to touch your nose to your knee, bring your head as far forward as you can, hold for the five count, and then let your head down. Increase the number of repetitions to ten on each side, and then proceed to Exercise VII.

Exercise VII
(SEE FIGURE 26)

The old-fashioned scissor exercise is still a favorite for improvement of stomach muscles as well as for thigh muscles. Women and men alike will enjoy the end benefit of tightening those thigh muscles without hurting their backs.

1. Lie on your back with knees bent and arms along your side but slightly away from your body to provide additional stability.

2. Bend and lift your thighs toward your body. Extend (straighten) your knees from this position. Your knees do not have to be perfectly straight; in fact, a slight bend in them is prefera-

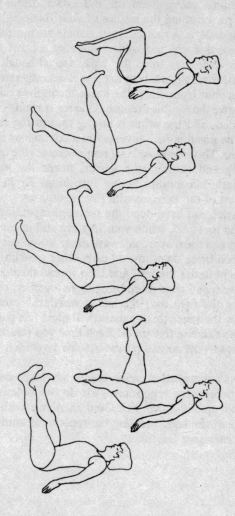

ble. Holding your legs in the air, pointing to the ceiling, move them up and down, from your hips, brushing the insides of your thighs as they pass. It is a motion very similar to the flutter kick that you use while swimming a crawl. The movement is from the hips, and although the knees are slightly bent to prevent excessive stretch on your hamstrings, the knees themselves do not move during this exercise. One leg is swung overhead, and the other is swung toward the floor. The positions are reversed in a continuous manner. This side-by-side motion resembles the opening and closing of a scissor, hence the name. Each full motion is one repetition. Begin this part of the exercise with five repetitions.

3. After you have done the required repetitions of the first part, while your legs are still in the air, spread them apart sideways as far as you can and then bring them toward each other, crossing the right under the left, and then spread them apart again and once more bring them together, crossing the right over the left (a wonderful exercise for the inner-thigh muscles). Repeat this part of the exercise five times. Each time you return the legs to the spread position is one repetition.

This is a sustained exercise, one in which you do not rest between each repetition. First do five repetitions with the up-and-down kick, and then five with the crossing of the legs. Increase the repetitions until you can do each part ten times.

Exercise VIII
(SEE FIGURE 27)

After Exercise VII, you need a little rest, and Exercise VIII is restful. This exercise is done lying on your stomach. From your standard position of lying on your back, turn over onto your stomach. Cross your arms in front of you, and rest your forehead on your arms so that you keep your head straight with some room to breathe.

If lying flat on your stomach causes pain in your lower back, a pillow beneath your pelvis will relieve the stress. This exercise is designed to strengthen your buttock muscles and stretch the muscles in front of your hip.

1. In the above position, lift your right leg from the floor with your knee straight. The actual lift is done from the hip. Keep your pelvis flat on the

EXERCISE VIII #27

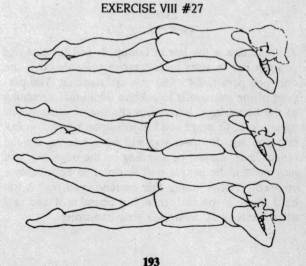

floor. There is a tendency to roll your pelvis to one side so that you can raise your leg higher. Avoid that tendency, because once you twist your pelvis with the leg up, you do not obtain the proper stretching of the muscles in front of the hip. Therefore, it is important to keep your pelvis flat. It really does not matter how high you lift the leg, as long as the front of the knee no longer touches the floor.

2. Once you have lifted your leg, hold it up for a count of five, and then let it down onto the floor. Relax a moment and repeat again for five repetitions. Then do the same exercise with your left leg.

While you're doing this exercise, your upper body should be relaxed. When you have achieved ten repetitions on each side, you are then ready to proceed to Exercise IX.

Exercise IX
(SEE FIGURE 28)

This exercise is the last in Group B, and for many of you the last in your back-exercise program. It is the only one performed while you are standing. The purpose of the exercise is to achieve additional stretching of the hamstrings. It requires the use of a chair, low table, desk, or other solid object upon which you can rest one leg. Because you will have one leg on the object, and you will be standing on the other leg, you may need to be near a wall in order to help balance yourself. If after trying this exercise, you find it too hard to do or painful, then just abandon it and rely upon Exercise IV to stretch your hamstrings.

1. Stand and face a hard chair or low table. Lift your right leg and place your heel on the top of the table. Turn your left leg so that your toes point sideways away from your body. (Hold on to the wall if you need balance support.)

2. Keeping your back upright and straight, place your right hand on your right thigh and slowly bend your left knee. As you bend your left knee, you lower your body. The right hand on the right knee helps to keep the right knee straight as your left knee bends. You will feel a pulling sensation in the back of your right thigh that indicates that you are stretching your hamstrings. The lower you bend the left leg, the greater the stretch on your right hamstrings. Remember, the right knee must be kept straight.

If you start with very tight hamstrings, moderate the amount of stretch you obtain by diminishing the bend of your left knee. As your hamstrings loosen, you can increase the bend of the left knee and stretch your right hamstring even further.

When you are able to bend the left knee a considerable distance and stretch the hamstring without feeling too much strain, you may then progress to a higher chair or table, which will increase the degree of stretch you can achieve. Remember to keep your back straight. Do *not* bend forward and try to touch your toes in this position. Runners and other athletes do this exercise that way, but they do not have back problems. As soon as you start to bend forward with this exercise, you are challenging your back, and unfortunately, it is a challenge that your back cannot rise to.

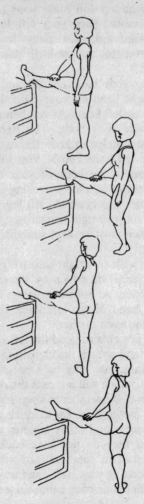

3. Sustain the stretch for a count of five. Do not bounce up and down. Straighten your left knee and repeat the exercise five times. Then do the same exercise for the left hamstrings, with the left heel on the table and bending your right knee.

Once you are able to do ten repetitions on each side, you will have completed the exercises in Group B. I would be entirely satisfied if you stopped here and did these nine exercises on a daily basis for the rest of your life. In fact, I would be ecstatic for you and for your back. However, there are some of you who feel they need more exercises, who want to become stronger and more fit. If that describes you, Group C exercises should help to satisfy that desire. I stress, though, that the first nine exercises are sufficient to keep your back healthy and to achieve the status of "no more aching back."

Group C Exercises

You may want to add any or all of these exercises to your back regime. These exercises are not so much additional exercises, but rather extensions of exercises that you are already doing. Please be careful with this group. They are more strenuous than the others, and not suitable for all backs. However, if you are able to perform them without pain, they can certainly further strengthen your muscles. With that caveat, I will describe the next four exercises.

Exercise 1 in Group C
(SEE FIGURE 29)

This exercise is done in conjunction with Exercise V, the modified sit-up.

1. After you have completed the modified sit-up, lock your hands behind your head, keep your knees bent, and then raise your head and shoulders off the floor.
2. Twist your right elbow toward your left knee and then your left elbow toward your right knee, and then drop your shoulders back to the floor. Repeat this exercise five times, and increase to ten or even twenty repetitions.

Exercise 2 in Group C
(SEE FIGURE 30)

Exercise 2 is just another adjunct to the other stomach exercises. It is strenuous and should be done with caution.

1. Lie on your back with your hands behind your head and legs outstretched on the floor with your feet together.
2. Lift up your head and shoulders with your hands behind your head, and hold that position. Then lift up your legs, with the knees straight. Hold your legs six inches off the floor, and keeping your knees stiff and straight, spread your legs wide apart and then bring them together. The combination of holding your head and shoulders up and at the same time lifting your legs, spreading them apart, and bringing them together is one of the most taxing of all stomach exercises. The lower back is protected during this exercise by remaining flat on the floor. Even so, this exercise may be too strenuous for you.
3. Holding the upper body off the floor, spread and bring your legs together five times. Then lower your back and legs, rest, and repeat five times.

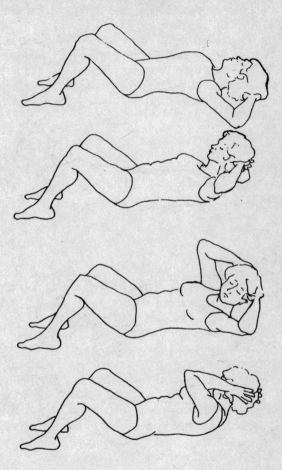

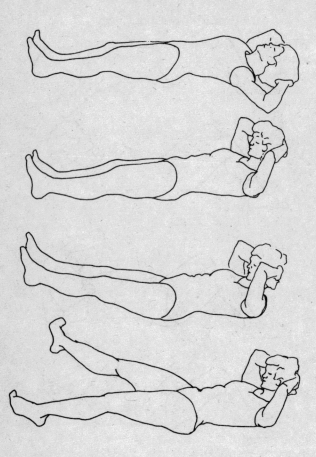

By performing the leg portion of the exercise ten times instead of five, you can increase the effectiveness of the exercise.

Exercises 3 and 4 in Group C

Whereas the first two exercises in this group concentrated on strengthening the stomach muscles, these last two exercises, 3 and 4, strengthen the muscles in your back. Again, they become an addition to the exercises you are already doing and should be done when you do the original exercise. In other words, keep the same sequential order that I outlined earlier.

Both Exercises 3 and 4 are done lying on your stomach in the position that I have described in Exercise VIII.

Exercise 3 in Group C
(SEE FIGURE 31)

After you have completed Exercise VIII, in which you lifted one leg at a time ten times, you can proceed with this exercise. Stay in the same prone position. Spread your legs apart, and lift them both simultaneously. Hold for a count of five and then lower. Repeat the exercise ten times.

Exercise 4 in Group C
(SEE FIGURE 32)

If you have managed the other exercises in this section, Exercise 4 will not be too hard for you. In this exercise, you hyperextend or arch your lower back. For most of this book, I have cautioned you not to arch or hyperextend your lower back. This motion can produce great pressure on your intervertebral disks, and if they are vulnerable can cause not only pain but

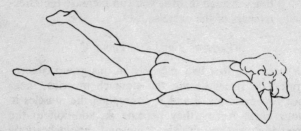

a risk of further disk herniation. However, at this moment in the sequence of your back-exercise program, your back should be strong and your damaged disk healed well enough to try this exercise. When you begin, do the hyperextension cautiously by not forcing the back into too much of an arc.

1. Lie on the floor on your stomach, and clasp your hands together behind your lower back.
2. Lift your head and shoulders up, and at the same time stretch your hands to behind your buttocks. Hold this position for a count of five, and then relax your head and shoulders but keep your hands behind your back. Slowly increase the number of repetitions to ten.

This last exercise is particularly helpful for a younger person with a round-shouldered posture and a curved upper back. If done regularly, this exercise can help to improve standing posture and also help prevent upper-spine deformities.

Now that you have read the complete list of exercises, a brief review may be helpful to get them into perspective.

4 IN C # 32

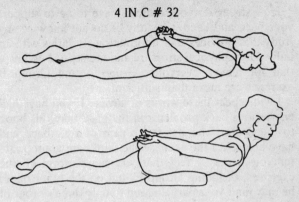

The first five exercises constitute Group A. This is the basic program for all backs. Exercise III, or the lumbar spine-twist exercise, may not be suitable for everyone. If it causes you pain, do not do it. The other four exercises will still be enormously helpful for you. Older people and those with particularly damaged or weak backs may only be able to do this first group of exercises.

The second group of exercises, Group B, consists of further strengthening movements. If you can add the four exercises in this group, or even one or two of them, your back will be even better. Again, remember that each of these has to be done carefully, and if any one of them is painful, do not do it.

Finally Group C exercises are the really tough ones. By virtue of being more strenuous to perform, they also build the strongest muscles. The Group C exercises are for those of you who feel that the other exercises are "too easy" and are not challenging enough. Even if you don't feel this way, however, if you can do these exercises (and have the time), Group C exercises can provide an even greater measure of support for your back.

How strong do your muscles have to be to support your back and keep it healthy? I do not know of any study that provides that information. It varies with an individual's physical structure and life-style. I do know that for almost everyone, Group A and Group B exercises are more than sufficient.

I will repeat these words of advice. If you have had any serious back problems in the past, take this book to the doctor who has taken care of your back and have him select the exercises he thinks are appropriate for you. He may feel that you can perform all the exercises, including Group C, but on the other hand, he may limit your participation to only three or four of the basic exercises. Your doctor is familiar with your particular back problem, and since there are so many different causes of back pain, it is wise to consult with him before beginning the exercise program.

CONCLUSION: NO MORE ACHING BACK

How do I summarize what it has taken an entire book to say? How can I avoid being overly repetitious? I must fail in both instances, because I cannot summarize this entire book in a few words, nor can I avoid repeating again what I consider the essential basis for obtaining and maintaining a healthy back. If repetition is the essence of teaching, then I have taught you well.

There are some specific thoughts and principles that I want you to remember. Foremost, you do not have to live with back pain forever. In most instances, you can control your back pain, although you may not cure it. The solution is in your hands in that you must practice good body habits, especially in regard to your back. Your posture, lifting, and carrying habits are all vitally important. The sooner you learn these good habits, the better your back will be.

Back exercises are essential ingredients for a healthy back. Whatever treatments you have had, and the different treatments are innumerable, nothing will be as important for your back as exercises. Even when back problems are caused or related to stress, exercises help both conditions, emotional and physical alike. There is no excuse for not doing your exercises. It requires determination, diligence, and intelligence—the latter because you should be smart enough to know how important and beneficial the exercises are for you.

When you are feeling really well, do not be lulled into a sense of false security and stop your exercises. I can guarantee that if you do stop the exercises, your back pain will come back to haunt you.

The Romans had a saying, "a healthy mind in a healthy body" (in Latin, *"mens sana in corpore sano"*). This book is about the health of your back, but if your body is healthy and in good condition, your back will be healthier too. The reverse is also true. If your back is in good shape, you can do more to promote a healthy body by exercising more freely and more vigorously. You can combine an aerobic-exercise program with your back exercises. There is no question that when your body is strong and healthy, your mind works better: Your attention span is longer, your retention of information is greater, your thought processes are quicker.

Keeping your body fit contributes to the health of your back and your mind.

The final message is that your body and your mind are of priceless value. They are irreplaceable for you. Although I have stressed the importance of your back and how to care for it in this book, I never lose sight of the entire person—you. As I have urged you to take care of your back, I also urge you to take care of yourself. Remember, as an individual, you are unique and priceless, so take good care of that body and mind.

I hope this book has been helpful to you. I send my best wishes for success, not only for achieving the status of "no more aching back," but also for all your endeavors.

Index

207

INDEX

INDEX

About the Author

LEON ROOT, M.D., is a well-known orthopedic surgeon in New York City. He is a full-time attending surgeon at the Hospital for Special Surgery where, among his other responsibilities, he is the director of Rehabilitation Medicine and of the Back School Program.